Not Tonight

Not Tonight

Migraine and the Politics of Gender and Health

JOANNA KEMPNER

THE UNIVERSITY OF CHICAGO PRESS CHICAGO AND LONDON

JOANNA KEMPNER is assistant professor of sociology and an affiliate of the Institute for Health, Health Care Policy, and Aging Research at Rutgers University.

The University of Chicago Press, Chicago 60637
The University of Chicago Press, Ltd., London
© 2014 by The University of Chicago
All rights reserved. Published 2014.
Printed in the United States of America
23 22 21 20 19 18 17 16 15 14   1 2 3 4 5

ISBN-13: 978-0-226-17901-8 (cloth)
ISBN-13: 978-0-226-17915-5 (paper)
ISBN-13: 978-0-226-17929-2 (e-book)
DOI: 10.7208/chicago/9780226179292.001.0001

Library of Congress Cataloging-in-Publication Data

Kempner, Joanna Leslie, author.
Not tonight : migraine and the politics of gender and health / Joanna Kempner.
pages cm
Includes bibliographical references and index.
ISBN 978-0-226-17901-8 (cloth : alk. paper)—ISBN 978-0-226-17915-5 (pbk. : alk. paper)—ISBN 978-0-226-17929-2 (e-book) 1. Migraine. 2. Migraine—Social aspects. 3. Headache—Social aspects. I. Title.
RC392.K45 2014
616.8'4912—dc23

2014004075

♾ This paper meets the requirements of ANSI/NISO Z39.48–1992 (Permanence of Paper).

TO MY PARENTS

Were headaches known in the Age of Gold; or, when the millennium shall prevail, will they cease to be? Certain it is, that in any state where there are secrets to conceal or pangs to dissemble, this convenient malady could no more be dispensed with than the most necessary article of attire. How could society possibly go on without the trite but inexhaustible excuse that—better than any soft answer—turns away wrath, and, for a while, at least, closes the mouth of the accuser, so that the accused, whether innocent or guilty, have time to breathe and brace themselves for the question, if it must needs ensue? There are people, I believe, who discourse quite eloquently on the advantages of gout; surely as many could be found ready to cry *Vive la migraine!*

GEORGE A. LAWRENCE, *Harper's New Monthly Magazine*, 1870

For the person in pain, so incontestably and unnegotiably present is it that "having pain" may come to be thought of as the most vibrant example of what it is to "have certainty," while for the other person it is so elusive that "hearing about pain" may exist as the primary model of what it is "to have doubt."

ELAINE SCARRY, *The Body in Pain*, 1985

Contents

Illustrations

Preface

My headaches began when I was five years old. A pediatrician diagnosed me with a "type A personality" and assured my parents that nothing could be done. My mother, herself debilitated by migraine, rejected his diagnosis. Thus began a long and frustrating quest for headache relief. By high school graduation, we had consulted at least a dozen or more health care providers, a group that included several general practitioners, a well-respected headache specialist, his clinic's psychiatrist, an acupuncturist, a massage therapist, an herbalist, as well as several chiropractors and physical therapists. Each relied on different diagnostic procedures, which were frustrating at best (a misread CAT scan indicated a rather alarming enlarged pituitary gland) and sometimes offensive (how often do patients get asked explicitly or otherwise whether their pain is real? Since pain is a sensation, isn't it always real?). Each had new treatments for me to try—anti-inflammatories and antidepressants, beta-blockers, muscle relaxants, painkillers, acupuncture, teas, diets, and homeopathic pills. I had needles embedded in my ears. I learned to meditate. I laid with my neck in traction. And I wished that one of my doctors would find a clear-cut biological abnormality that could explain my pain. A tumor might be removed, I reasoned.

In college, I managed these headaches with a firm commitment to denial and a cocktail of prescription painkillers and muscle relaxants. The medications never relieved the pain, but they helped me sleep or, sometimes, just laugh it off. Needless to say, plans were canceled and classes missed. Eventually, I learned that my headaches were migraines. Like so many other people with migraine (a disorder that experts always refer to in the singular), I would find myself vomiting in an emergency room, hoping that nobody would treat me like a drug addict who invents pain in exchange for narcotics. Entering the workforce posed more problems. I worried about telling coworkers that I had migraine—I wanted them to think of me as reliable. But I missed so many days that I decided to explain that I had chronic migraine to potential employers. I thought it was better to be up front than fired later.[1] Most showed compassion, but I found it hard to call out of work sick. After all, doesn't everyone have headaches?

The answer is yes—almost everyone gets headaches from time to time. Headaches are one of the most common symptoms in the population—over 95 percent of the population is estimated to have a headache at some point in their lifetime.[2] As a result, almost everyone has well-intentioned, often contradictory, and always ill-advised recommendations for those who have serious headache disorders: drink more water, take two aspirin, do yoga, meditate, seek acupuncture and Chinese medicine, alter your diet, take regular exercise, do not exercise strenuously, take vitamins, take herbs, use heat, use ice, use nothing, relax, or, most annoyingly, "just think about something else." Some of these recommendations can help some of the time, but most are useless to the person in serious pain.[3] While headache is the primary symptom of most serious headache disorders, it is not the defining symptom (surprisingly, migraine can exist without pain), nor is the head pain comparable to the garden-variety headaches that most people experience.

Like so many other pain conditions, headache disorders are invisible. They are also difficult to describe to the uninitiated. The symptoms that accompany headache disorders—like head pain, visual auras, and sensitivity to sound—are difficult to measure and easy for practitioners to discount because they lack an objective marker of distress that can confirm their existence. Headache disorders provide no outward signs: people with headache disorders have no broken bones, no casts or slings, no limps, blood tests, or X-rays to point to when they hurt. Even someone with a severely disabling headache disorder can appear healthy upon physical examination. As a result, I often felt that each doctor's appointment was a test of my credibility. I worked on the best ways to convey my symptoms without appearing hyperbolic or, worse, hypochondriacal.

Doctors rely on patient reports of symptoms to diagnose migraine and other headache disorders. As one might imagine, we are not easy patients. We are repeat visitors and we are frustrated and frustrating. When objective tests fail to show an organic pathology, when drugs fail to produce their intended effect, when recommended diets, exercises, and lifestyle changes fail to lessen the frequency or duration of the headaches, it may be hard to escape that nagging question: how much does this pathology exist within the mind of the patient?

Doctor visits are further complicated by what Judy Segal, a scholar of rhetoric, has described as the ghosts of patients past. Physicians, she argues, already have a "mental cast of characters" that they anticipate when meeting a headache patient.[4] The clinical encounter, therefore, is truly a performance, as people with headache disorders attempt to persuade their doctor that they are not the expected "hysterical woman," "malinger," "hypochondriac," or "drug seeker" but a person with a legitimate problem. Women are more prone to such interpretations and report they must "work hard" to present themselves as credible patients.[5] This often translates into an effort to carefully control gender displays. Nobody wants to be viewed as a whiny, weak-willed girl. This is a challenging balance. Patients wonder how to be assertive, while conveying a sense of just how badly they hurt. Even with these efforts, patients report that they are "met with skepticism and lack of comprehension," and that they feel "rejected, ignored and . . . belittled."[6]

So one may imagine my surprise and delight when I turned on the radio in 2000 and heard a prominent headache specialist, Stephen Silberstein, the director of the famed Jefferson Headache Center in Philadelphia, tell his audience: "We used to believe that migraine was a disorder of neurotic women, whose blood vessels dilated and they couldn't face up to life. We now know that migraine is a disorder of the brain."[7] Eureka! I was thrilled that the medical establishment had finally confirmed what I had known my entire life: migraine is, in fact, a "real" disorder. But I began to have doubts about Silberstein's declaration when the first caller rang into the show. He began, "I have been suffering in retrospect since about the age of twelve or thirteen, although I have to tell you when you mentioned it's a neurological condition, it sounds a little scarier than what I had thought." The host of the show asked Silberstein to respond to the caller's fear: "He hears the word neurobiological and it scares him. Should he be scared? Is that a scary word?" Silberstein responded authoritatively, "It means it's a real disorder, it's not something in your head. It means it's a disorder of the brain tissue itself."

Reflecting on this moment instantly reminds me how pleasantly surprised I was that someone was taking migraine seriously. Silberstein's confidence that migraine was real suggested a possible end to a lifetime of alienation in the clinic. I wanted to believe in Silberstein's vision: that science had offered an objective, gender-neutral model of migraine, one that no longer considers migraine to be "a disorder of neurotic women." But I was also intrigued by the caller's ambivalence about the word "neurological." A disease meant that something was truly wrong with him. What I had heard as good news (i.e., I am not crazy), the caller had interpreted as bad news (i.e., he has a disorder of the brain tissue). The caller's anxious question swiftly reminded me that both disease and theories about its causes are awash with multiple and often contradictory meanings. I wondered at what point I began interpreting "bad news" as "good news" and how ironic it was that we often prefer to have a neurological disease than be diagnosed with something that brings our rationality into question. And then I wondered: if I thought it was better to have a neurological disease and this shaped my thinking about the brain, how do these same cultural ideas affect an expert like Stephen Silberstein? How do our entrenched ideas about mind, body, gender, and legitimacy shape what *he* believes about migraine?

Over the years, these questions turned into an examination of the relationship between gender and the politics of legitimacy in headache medicine. For example, if biomedicine has discovered that migraine is "real," why does it remain so easy to ignore, dismiss, and delegitimate? Has the "discovery" of the brain in migraine really erased the idea of the hysterical patient that is so deeply embedded in doctor-patient interactions about pain? In this book, I argue that the recent biomedicalization of migraine is not powerful enough to erase centuries of sexism in culture and in medicine. If anything, the transformation of migraine from a disorder of the mind to a disease of the brain has reified some of the same stultified ideas about gender that always made life difficult for both men and women in pain. The result has important implications for how we understand whose pain and suffering is taken seriously and whose is ignored on an individual level, at the clinic, in the annals of medical journals, and by policy makers.

C. Wright Mills famously wrote that the sociological imagination begins when we think about our personal troubles as public issues.[8] Taking this to heart, I spent eleven years following headache researchers, patient advocates, and pharmaceutical representatives from conference to conference, analyzing textbooks, medical articles, promotional materials, advertisements, Internet forums, and advocacy efforts. As a scholar, I have learned a great deal about headache disorders and their treatment. As a patient-scholar, I approach this subject from a personal perspective, which I am sure has colored what I have chosen to write about.[9] My own experience with migraine serves as a standard against which I inevitably use to filter all that I read, hear, and learn about headaches. Admittedly, this grants me a subjective position shaped by my multiple encounters with the medical system, skepticisms about certain treatments that worsened my disorder, and optimistic feelings about others that made me feel better. Moreover, my disorder has not remained stable throughout this study. When I began, my migraines were a minor irritation. But they worsened with time. For years, I have had chronic migraine, meaning that I experience a headache more days than I do not. The list of treatments tried has grown to include new preventives, diets, nerve blocks, Botox, and even multiple days spent in outpatient and inpatient infusion centers, where nurses deliver strong medications through an IV or PICC line. Treatments have had varying levels of success.

This book offers the kind of analysis that could only come from an insider with an embodied knowledge of migraine. Pain comes without a voice. The best way to learn about the cultural politics of legitimacy in migraine is through the body—to *feel* what it is like to experience a disorder that few view as an actual problem. My position as an insider provides tangible benefits. Having migraine helped me develop rapport with patient advocates and headache specialists—the former because I could relate to their experiences and the latter because I could speak to them both as a colleague and a patient. My insider status also aided analysis of data. I understand medical discourse on migraine from the inside out. I can tell you how bare diagnostic criteria fail to capture the nuances of the various pains I feel upon waking. I understand the frustration of multiple doctors' appointments, prescriptions, and ineffective treatments. I have taken most of the new drugs on the market and many of the old versions, too. I understand how challenging it is to move through the world when something as lovely as perfume or a glass of wine becomes a veritable landmine, ready to trigger a torrent of pain. My body became a fieldnote.[10] So my analysis proceeds with one foot in the medical world, one foot in sociology, and my head riddled with migraines.

But as I argue throughout this book, I am not the only one in the headache community who has an interest in shaping the discourse surrounding migraine. All researchers, especially headache specialists, have vested interests that shape both what is studied and what is obscured. One study revealed that most neurologists who seek additional training in headache have migraine themselves.[11] The same is true of the headache specialists who run clinics and produce research on the topic. Some of them told me that having migraine provides them with added insight into the disorder. Or they make the claim that having migraine allows them to form better rapport with their patients. This seems sensible—patients who worry about the credibility of their symptoms would surely welcome treatment form someone who also has a headache disorder. But none of these headache specialists ever write about their personal experience with headache disorders in articles or books. They believe that the scientific process renders their own experience with headache irrelevant, that their knowledge (and, indeed, the best knowledge) is disembodied and fully removed from the knower. This kind of objective knowledge is best, it is believed, because it offers a knowledge set that is universal and transcendent in nature and scope, in a way in which embodied knowledge can never be. I disagree that the producer of knowledge or, more importantly, the context in which this knowledge is produced, can ever truly disappear. Indeed, the objectivity of science depends upon the suppression of the knower.[12] In contrast, feminist science studies argues that self-reflexivity can make for better knowledge production, since logic, rationality, and even objectivity are all filtered through one's personal experience, local workplaces, and cultural milieu. In that spirit, my embodied experiences as a fieldworker and as a person with migraine are woven throughout this text.

There are, however, interests that can have a pernicious effect on scientific knowledge production. As I discuss in chapter 4, the headache research community is supported, in large part, by private dollars from the pharmaceutical industry. Without these funds, headache specialists would conduct far less research, publish fewer articles, and organize much less elaborate conferences. Most leaders in headache medicine earn at least part of their income from the pharmaceutical industry. This close economic dependency is troubling because it suggests an overriding corporate interest in the shape and trajectory of headache specialists' research agendas. The rhetoric of objectivity may be de rigueur in medicine, but this does nothing to alter these vested interests. Mine are simply made explicit.

Finally, a warning to those who are searching for a self-help guide on how to live with headache disorders. My interests are cultural (not medical). Many excellent books describe the neurophysiology of migraine, review treatment options, or teach patients how to advocate on behalf of their own health. My goal is different. I aim to understand the cultural medium in which researchers, patient advocates, and pharmaceutical companies understand and disseminate knowledge about migraine and other headache disorders. While I will not be providing a how-to guide of life in pain, I do hope to clarify the cultural landscape that colors our collective experience of living with headache. I don't pretend that this will provide any relief to pain and yet, at the same time, I agree with Siri Hustvedt, a novelist who often writes about her own migraines, when she says that "intellectual curiosity about one's own illness is certainly born of a desire for mastery."[13] Perhaps a greater cultural understanding of our bodies can help, in some tiny part, alleviate the greater suffering of those in pain.

Acknowledgments

A great many people in the headache community have dedicated their professional life to finding treatments and, ultimately, a cure for migraine and cluster headache. Their work is crucial for those of us who live in pain. I owe a particular debt to the people who shared their time and insight with me over the past few years. Richard B. Lipton, Elizabeth Loder, Steven Peroutka, and Robert Shapiro provided steady encouragement and constructive feedback. I am especially grateful to William B. Young, whose enthusiasm for this project often exceeded my own. He read many of the chapters in this book and provided incisive comments and insights into the field. As my headache doctor, he also worked tirelessly to help me feel better. I am equally grateful to the headache advocates who welcomed me into their communities, including Catherine Charrett-Dykes, Megan Oltman, Teri Robert, and Kary Shannon. Thanks, also, to Amrita Bhowmick and the Migraine.com team, for offering me a space to practice public sociology.

Research for this book began at the University of Pennsylvania, where the Department of Sociology and the Center for Bioethics supported my work. I am tremendously lucky to have been mentored by Charles L. Bosk, who guided my work with compassion, generosity, and brilliant insight. I was the grateful beneficiary of the kindness and wisdom of Susan Lindee and Robert Aronowitz, who taught me how to think like a historian as well as a sociologist. Jason Schnittker provided excellent feedback and support and Jon Merz offered research opportunities that allowed me to grow as a scholar.

At the University of Michigan, I had the good fortune to work as a Robert Wood Johnson Scholar in Health Policy Research. Paula Lantz and Mike Chernew directed this fantastic program, which provided me with time and resources to expand my research. I also benefited from frequent, spirited discussions with Renee Anspach, John DiNardo, James House, and Jonathan Metzl. Afterward, Betsy Armstrong welcomed me to the Center for Health and Wellbeing at Princeton University. She is a tremendously generous mentor and friend, and she provided me with intellectual and emotional support. I will always be grateful for the time that she spent down in the trenches with me—this manuscript spread over a large conference table—trying to work through some of its more intransigent problems. Over these years, I enjoyed the collegiality, collective wisdom, and humor of Neal Caren, Amy Love Collins, Brian Goesling, Amie Hess, Jeff Hornstein, Margot Jackson, Mireille Jacobson, Julie Kmec, Catherine Lee, Helen Lee, Susan Markens, Joanie Mazelis, Heather Royer, Bhaven Sampat, Olga Shevchenko, and Tyson Smith. Thanks also to Tania Jenkins, who provided important feedback.

This book was midwifed into existence in the Department of Sociology at Rutgers University. I am very lucky to work in a deeply intellectual and collegial environment. I have received more than my fair share of encouragement and sound advice from all of my colleagues, especially Debby Carr, Karen Cerulo, Chip Clarke, Phaedra Daipha, Judy Gerson, Allan Horwitz, Laurie Krivo, Paul McLean, Pat Roos, Kristen Springer, and Arlene Stein. Julie Philips and Eviatar Zerubavel helped me negotiate the tenure track, reading my work and providing me with invaluable professional advice. Lisa Iorillo gracefully helped me navigate the vast Rutgers bureaucracy. Catherine Lee talked me through innumerable intellectual, professional, and personal challenges, and made sure I was fed and having a good time. Rutgers University is an exceptional place to be a medical sociologist and feminist scholar. David Mechanic and the Institute for Health, Health Care Policy and Aging Research amply supported my research. Members of the department's workshop on Gender, Difference and Inequality read an early draft of a book chapter and provided comments that helped shape a central argument running through the text. I also benefited from a fellowship provided by the Center for Cultural Analysis.

Many people have read and commented on multiple drafts of this work. In addition to many of those mentioned above, I am very grateful for the expertise, kindness, and constructive criticism of Rene Almeling, Linda Blum, Laura Carpenter, Sejal Patel, Jennifer Reich, and Audra Wolfe, each of whom offered me thoughtful advice on how to make this a better book. Of course, any errors that remain are mine.

For the generous support of the research and writing of this book, I thank the University of Pennsylvania's Otto and Gertrude K. Pollak Research Fellowship, the Robert Wood Johnson Foundation, Princeton University's Center for Health and Wellbeing, Rutgers University's Institute for Health, Health Care Policy and Aging Research, and Rutgers University's National Science Foundation RU-Fair Lifecycle grant. I also thank the College of Physicians of Philadelphia, the Wellcome Library, and the Medical Center Archives of New York–Presbyterian/Weill Cornell for generously providing access to their collections.

Portions of chapter 4 were published previously as "Gendering the Migraine Market: Do Gendered Representations of Illness Matter?" *Social Science and Medicine* 63, no. 8 (2006): 1986–97. A version of chapter 5 was published as "Uncovering the Man in Medicine: Lessons Learned from a Case Study of Cluster Headache," *Gender and Society* 20, no. 5 (2006): 632–56, doi: 10.1177/0891243206290720.

A close group of old friends deserves my deepest gratitude for putting up with me over the years: Erica Benjamin, Amy Chao, Mara Cooper, Hollace Detwiler, Jivey Rivas, and Shelby Siegel. I admire them for their passion, intelligence, creativity, and wit.

Many thanks to my extended family, the Drurys, who kept my spirits up by taking me on delightful summer holidays and providing me with loads of nieces and nephews to dote upon. Melissa Stone became my confidante and advisor. The Kempners provided an untold amount of emotional support, but I also used them as research assistants as often as I could. Evan Kempner wrote a software program that scraped pharmaceutical websites for images. Michelle Kempner helped code these advertisements and provided technical assistance. My mother, Ruth Kempner, is part of my inspiration for this book, and she also served as a reliable sounding board for emerging ideas. My father, Jim Kempner, read every word of this manuscript. His edits were quick, sharp, and always pushed me to tell a better story.

I couldn't have finished this book without Joe Drury. He spent countless hours helping me work through difficult problems, and always had the good sense to tell me when I had to go back to the drawing board. He made me laugh, gave me reasons to take breaks, and took care of me when I was sick. Our best times, however, are spent with Noah, who brings us joy every day.

Abbreviations

(AHDA)	Alliance for Headache Disorders Advocacy
(AAN)	American Academy of Neurology
(AASH)	American Association for the Study of Headache
(ACHE)	American Council for Headache Education
(AHMA)	American Headache and Migraine Association
(AHDA)	American Headache Disorders Alliance
(AHS)	American Headache Society
(DSM)	Diagnostic and Statistical Manual of Mental Disorders
(FDA)	Food and Drug Administration
(GSK)	GlaxoSmithKline
(ICHD)	International Classification of Headache Disorders
(IHC)	International Headache Congress
(IHS)	International Headache Society
(MAGNUM)	Migraine Awareness Group: A National Understanding for Migraineurs
(NHF)	National Headache Foundation
(NINDS)	National Institute of Neurological Disorders and Stroke
(NIH)	National Institutes of Health
(NYHF)	New York Headache Foundation
(OUCH)	Organization for the Understanding of Cluster Headache
(PhRMA)	Pharmaceutical Research and Manufacturers of America
(WHA)	World Headache Alliance
(WHO)	World Health Organization

Introduction

Scottie Pippen, a basketball player with the Chicago Bulls, had an extraordinary career. Alongside teammate Michael Jordan, he led the Bulls to six National Basketball Association (NBA) championship titles, played in the 1996 US Olympic "Dream Team," and was named an NBA all-star for seven years. So great were his achievements that the Chicago Bulls retired his jersey number, "33," when he left the game. But a shadow hangs over Pippen's otherwise remarkable career. To this day, whenever sports fans and commentators talk about or interview Pippen, they inevitably turn to the migraine that kept him from helping the Bulls win the 1990 Eastern Conference Championship.

The migraine that defined so much of his career came on during the seventh and final game of the playoffs. If they won, the Bulls would have played in their first-ever NBA Finals. Pippen stayed in for 42 minutes (of a total 48 minutes), but he turned in one of his worst performances, hitting only 1 of 10 attempted shots. The Bulls lost 93–74.

Reporters slammed Pippen's performance immediately after the game. In interviews, Pippen blamed a migraine, which he said made it difficult for him to distinguish the distance between himself and his teammates. In a June 11, 1990, article, Mike Weber, a writer for the *Sporting News*, asked whether Pippen was "so nervous that he brought on the physical affliction himself." The Bulls' trainer fueled his speculation by suggesting that Pippen was in fact affected by stress: "If you get excited because of the adrenaline in your system, it can have an effect on the vision. . . . I think that's why he got the blurry vision." Pippen disagreed: "I wasn't nervous at all. I have been through tough games similar to this one, and nothing happened. I tried to play through [the migraine]." His objections were largely ignored, despite the fact that migraines often do cause visual disturbances.

The story broke another way: Pippen had "choked." Although he continued to perform as an all-star, he never fully escaped the nickname: "Scottie 'Not Tonight, I Have a Headache' Pippen."[1]

In 1990, many doctors would likely have agreed with sportswriters who attributed Pippen's migraines to nerves. Most of the medical establishment still thought of migraine as a psychosomatic condition that manifested itself in people with controlling personalities and was exacerbated by stressful situations. By the new millennium, however, fMRI brain scans, pharmaceutical interventions, and genetic research had helped redefine migraine as a neurobiological disorder. Researchers disproved the existence of a "migraine personality." Although there is still much to be learned about its causes, migraine is now believed to be a biological disease like any other—a fact that advocates advertise in an effort to legitimate and destigmatize migraine.

Nevertheless, public figures who admit to having migraine remain subject to ridicule. Take, for example, the case of philanthropist and political spouse Cindy McCain. After many years struggling with debilitating chronic migraine, McCain decided to become a spokesperson, throwing her full support and considerable political connections behind efforts to advocate for migraine research. She talked to reporters about her own experiences and delivered a keynote speech to the 2009 International Headache Congress. The *New Yorker* responded by mocking her activism for migraine. In a segment titled the "Not Tonight Dept.," the magazine listed migraine as one of many ailments that McCain had already complained about, including a sprained wrist obtained "when a supporter [of her husband's presidential campaign] 'very vigorously' pumped her right hand." Noting that "everything about her seemed lemony," the *New Yorker* described McCain's commentary as "astringent."[2] McCain came off as an overprivileged socialite whining about an insignificant discomfort. Migraine remains an opportunity to make jokes about moral character despite its designation as a "real" neurobiological disorder in contemporary biomedical knowledge.

Of course, professional ballplayers and philanthropists are not typical Americans. But their struggle with migraine symptoms, disability, and the stigma attached to it closely parallels the experience of approximately thirty-six million of their fellow citizens. Take Marilyn Barton, for example. Barton, a woman in her thirties, has dealt with chronic migraine since childhood, and she feels both "crippled" and "embarrassed" by migraine:

> It's depressing because you—you feel crippled, but it's not in a very visible way, and you always wonder if people think you're just sort of a very whiny person. And you are. You sort of—I can't stand—I think to myself, "God, I can't stand myself." . . . It is embarrassing to have to say you're leaving work because you have a headache, even when you say it's a migraine, because at least, I guess, I feel like my co-workers see it as a way of sort of slinking out of work or a very silly excuse.[3]

Marilyn Barton, Cindy McCain, and Scottie Pippen are very different people, but they are linked by the shared experience of delegitimation. All three are confronted with others' skepticism regarding the reality of their symptoms and the extent of their pain.

Not Tonight examines how migraine can simultaneously disrupt so many lives and continue to be questioned and trivialized by the culture at large. Why do some kinds of pain generate deep sympathy and hefty economic investment, while other kinds are ignored? Why do we privilege and even praise some sorts of pain, while others are perceived as unimportant? Why does some people's pain matter more than others? Why, for example, are endurance athletes who suffer for their successes celebrated as heroes (even as they choose and train for such pain), while people who live in chronic pain (also a feat of endurance, and one for which there is no finish line) are dismissed as "whiny" or weak willed? Sometimes, a particularly severe headache attracts attention (and sympathy) as a symptom of something more serious, like an aneurysm or a stroke. But much of the time, migraine is seen as a "silly excuse." That the medical recasting of migraine as a neurobiological disorder has not altered this cultural configuration highlights the social contests that surround migraine's legitimacy and cultural significance.

As much as we understand pain to be the ultimate private experience, one endured by the individual alone, the identification and treatment of pain occur within a context of rich and often conflicting cultural formulations.[4] Pain can be victimizing or a source of strength, rooted in the body or a figment of the imagination, soul-destroying or transformative. Our perception of migraine depends on its positioning within these binaries. Moreover, pain is difficult to communicate effectively. Pain is invisible, impossible to quantify objectively, and rarely causes fatalities.[5] Pain interrupts mind/body dualisms in ways that can make it hard for others to understand.

In *Not Tonight*, I especially focus on how gender overdetermines how pain is understood. Gender, I argue, gets written into the way we talk about, understand, and make policies for people who have headache disorders. I uncover the surprising ways that biomedicine rearticulates and reifies some of our most crass assumptions about men and women, even as scientists explicitly work toward creating objective, gender-neutral knowledge. This book also shows the extent to which people with migraine and a related disorder, cluster headache, are willing to embrace these gendered assumptions, as long as their symptoms are legitimated as real and serious. This book additionally investigates how the pharmaceutical industry profits from portraying migraine as a lifestyle condition of white, middle-class women, even as these representations subvert well-intentioned efforts to diagnose and treat people in pain. Ultimately, this book explores the role that gender plays in mediating which forms of pain are legitimated and which forms of pain are not.

The Migraine Experience

Migraine is an incredibly common experience, affecting about 12 percent of the adult population each year.[6] Women are disproportionately affected, making up about three-quarters of those with migraine, meaning that 18 percent of adult American women have migraine. However, this sex difference does not appear until puberty. An equal number of boys and girls have migraine: 7 percent.[7] Most research attributes the sex difference that emerges to hormones or sex-linked genetic transmission.[8]

Migraine also appears to be more prevalent among whites than blacks. An estimated 9.8 percent of blacks have migraine (versus 12.4 percent of whites). More blacks than whites (6.1 percent versus 4.25 percent), however, have what is called “probable migraine”—a diagnosis in which an individual’s symptoms fit most, but not all, of the guidelines for migraine.[9] In addition, like many other diseases, migraine is more prevalent among people with low incomes.[10] However, there is little research investigating epidemiological differences in migraine by race and class, so it is not clear whether these disparities ought to be attributed to inadequacies in epidemiological survey data collection, like racial differences in symptom reporting, or social factors that make whites and the working class more susceptible to migraine. Nevertheless, these figures suggest that social and biological factors both contribute to migraine. Unfortunately, almost all research on migraine focuses on biological correlates. Very little discourse invokes racial or socioeconomic disparities. If anything, migraine is presumed to be a disorder of white, middle-class women.

Migraine is a spectrum disorder, meaning that those who have the diagnosis experience a wide range of symptoms to varying extents. Although headache is the most common symptom associated with migraine, migraine attacks include more than head pain. Diagnostic criteria also include nausea, vomiting, and hypersensitivity to light or sound. (Diagnostic criteria as outlined in the International Classification of Headache Disorders-III [ICHD-III] is included in appendix A.) Many people with migraine experience a "prodrome," which is a preheadache phase that includes such symptoms as food cravings, constipation, and fatigue. About 20 percent of people with migraine also experience an "aura," which follows the prodrome but precedes the headache and involves a variety of neurological symptoms like visual, auditory, or olfactory hallucinations; tingling in the extremities; difficulty in finding words; confusion; vertigo; hypersensitivity to feel and touch; or even partial paralysis. Typically, a headache follows, but migraine can also occur without headache—such migraine attacks are sometimes referred to as "migraine equivalents" and include a constellation of symptoms that denote the typical characteristics of migraine with the exception of headache. This manifestation is common in children, who may receive a diagnosis of migraine upon presenting with cyclical bouts of nausea. The "postdrome" follows the headache and can include such symptoms as depression or euphoria, fatigue, poor concentration, or cognitive impairment. Migraine and its variants are considered to be primary headache conditions, which means the symptoms constitute their own disorder, as opposed to a secondary headache disorder that would be caused by an identifiable underlying medical problem like a brain tumor or aneurysm.

Most people who have migraine are on the mild end of the spectrum; they might experience one to three headache days per month and lose some functionality as a result of symptoms. But about a quarter experience severe levels of disability associated with their symptoms.[11] One to 3 percent of American adults are estimated to have "chronic migraine," in which intermittent migraines progressively become more frequent—people with chronic migraine experience at least fifteen or more headache days a month for at least three months in a row.[12] To put these numbers in perspective, epilepsy affects 2.1 million Americans. Autism affects half a million Americans.[13] Chronic migraine affects 2.4 to 7.1 million American adults.

People with migraine frequently say that you have to experience a migraine to really understand how bad it can be. The headache typically associated with migraine lasts anywhere between four and seventy-two hours. The pain ranges from moderate to severe, but even moderately painful migraines can be significantly disabling.[14] People with migraine describe how the pain "made sleep impossible . . . [and] cause[d] severe bodily pain, tiredness, sweating, and lack of memory."[15] Migraine limits individuals' ability not only to work and "fulfill their real potential" but also often their ability to "get out of bed."[16] Cindy McCain compared her chronic migraines to her husband Senator John McCain's experience of torture in Vietnam: "Being tied to a chair for four days. I can't imagine how unbearable that pain must have been, but yeah, I can, because a migraine may come close."[17] The suffering is such that essayist Joan Didion wrote: "That no one dies of migraine seems, to someone deep into an attack, an ambiguous blessing."[18]

Studies show that people with migraine do not on the whole see migraine as an episodic condition consisting of individual attacks; they see it instead as a chronic disorder that affects their quality of life all the time.[19] Having unpredictable migraine attacks makes it difficult to make plans. Regular work hours can be problematic or impossible to maintain. Any number of triggers can set off the chain of events that ultimately leads to a migraine attack: hormonal changes, weather fronts, altitude, stress, alcohol, odors, monosodium glutamate (MSG), high blood pressure, changes in sleep patterns, or physical exertion. Sometimes the migraine happens immediately, sometimes days later. Management of triggers lends itself to an ascetic lifestyle, stripped free of caffeine and alcohol, physical exertion, late nights out, perfume, and foods as varied as bananas, citrus, gluten, and Chinese cuisine (all rumored to trigger migraines). Preventive pharmaceutical treatments can take their toll on daily lives, as well. The best migraine preventives only reduce frequency of headache symptoms by 50 percent for 50 percent of those who take them. Moreover, these drugs often come with difficult-to-tolerate side effects. (The primary drug used for migraine prevention, Topamax (topiramate), has been nicknamed "dopamax," because it often causes cognitive troubles for users.)

Alongside migraine's symptoms, delegitimation seems to be a fundamental component of the migraine experience. The doubt surrounding the ontology of migraine—what it is exactly—is so infectious that people sometimes come to question their own experience of the disorder. Jeff Tweedy, the lyricist, lead singer, and guitarist of the critically acclaimed rock band Wilco, had such severe migraines that, during shows, he would vomit into a bucket that he kept just offstage. Still, he writes that "as migraine sufferer you begin to doubt yourself. . . . There were a lot times when I wondered, 'Am I really getting a migraine or am I just dreading what I have to do and because of that starting to work myself up in to lather [*sic*]?' "[20] Others express similar doubts. Kerrie Smyres, a headache advocate whose symptoms are disabling enough to keep her from paid employment, regularly posts entries on her blog *The Daily Headache* about whether she is proactive enough in seeking rehabilitative treatment, whether her pain is as bad as she thinks it is, and even whether she has brought this pain on herself. This is partly why people with migraine report remarkably high levels of internalized stigma.[21] People worry when they cannot fulfill their end of the so-called sick role, an implicit social contract in which sick people are given leave of their everyday duties, as long as they adhere to certain rules like seeking appropriate medical help and working hard to get better.[22] But these obligations are difficult to meet when there is so little effective treatment. Moreover, culture is a powerful medium through which we experience our identity. If, as sociologist Charles Horton Cooley argued, we form our sense of self through the edict "I am who I think you think I am," then ongoing cultural narratives equating headaches with weakness are constantly operating to create insecure and diminished selves.[23]

Headaches strike a central feature of personhood. The head is an area of particular cultural sensitivity in which to experience pain. In a modern Western landscape fundamentally shaped by the Cartesian dictum "I think, therefore I am," the head is often considered the center of personality. The head houses the brain and can be used to describe the seat of the faculty or reason, as in "she calculated it in her head," or as a metaphor for mental ability or aptitude: "he has a good head for strategy." The head is also used to indicate authority; a person who leads or is in charge is referred to as "head of the organization," and political leaders are often called "heads of state." The "head of the household" sits at the "head of the table." The head is so essential in Western understandings of personhood that an individual's existence or job is often reduced to the synecdoche of the head—"it cost him his head."

Both migraine patients and their physicians struggle to sort out whether these head problems are indicative of a more serious underlying pathology or the result of anxieties, strong emotions, or other psychological factors. Headache patients frequently wonder out loud whether they might have a brain tumor, which is an unlikely possibility.[24] But when doctors cannot locate an organic cause of their symptoms, patients may fear that the pain is literally "all in their head." This anxiety need not be fed directly by the doctor (although physicians do sometimes mistake headache disorders for psychological distress). The mixture of self-doubt and fear creates a potent form of psychic suffering.[25]

Sadly, the worst fears of people with migraine are often realized when they enter a medical clinic. Physicians are too often skeptical when it comes to headache disorders and the people who have them. Despite migraine's designation as a "real" neurobiological disorder, people with migraine still struggle to be taken seriously at the clinic. Neurologists view headache disorders as an undesirable condition to treat—a disturbing attitude, given that neurology is the specialty that, by and large, is responsible for providing care for those with difficult-to-treat headache disorders. A survey of neurologists, commissioned by the American Academy of Neurology (AAN), found that nearly half (49 percent) "felt that headache patients were more time consuming" and a third (35 percent) found them "more emotionally draining" than other patients. Half perceived headache patients "as having more psychiatric problems than other patients." And a quarter (24 percent) of those surveyed felt that headache patients were motivated to maintain their disability.[26]

In addition, public response to headache disorders has been weak, at best. Federal funding for migraine research, for example, is radically inconsistent with its economic and social burden. According to the World Health Organization (WHO), migraine is the nineteenth-most significant cause of disability worldwide and the twelfth-most significant cause of disability worldwide for women.[27] The economic loss is huge, especially since migraine is most common among people between the ages of twenty-five and forty-four, when they are most likely to participate in the workforce. As a result, American employers lose more than $31 billion per year in productivity.[28] And yet, in recent years, the National Institutes of Health (NIH) has only increased its spending on headache-related research to $20–$25 million.[29] Most of this research funding goes toward migraine. Other headache disorders, like chronic daily headache and cluster headache, receive almost no public funding at all.

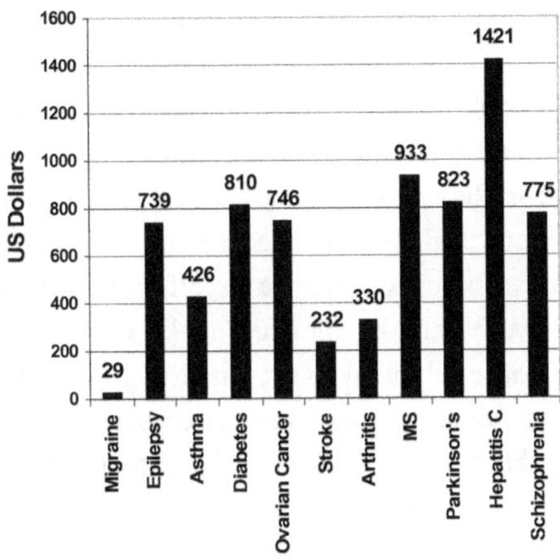

FIGURE I.1 2007 NIH Funding per DALY (Disability-Adjusted Life Years). Data from Schwendt and Shapiro, "Funding of Research on Headache Disorders by the National Institutes of Health," 167.

This figure is deeply out of sync with funding for other diseases, especially considering the burden that migraine causes. For example, migraine accounts for three times as many years lived with disability (or Disability-Adjusted Life Years, DALYs, as the WHO calls them) as epilepsy, but epilepsy generally receives about $105 million per year. Hepatitis C receives about $108 million from the NIH, even though it causes less than 20 percent of the disability that migraine creates.[30] This discrepancy can be seen in figure I.1.[31] The dearth of federal funding means that almost all headache-disorders research is funded by the pharmaceutical industry.

The Legitimacy Deficit

Headache disorders are among a number of contested illnesses, including chronic fatigue syndrome, attention deficit disorder, fibromyalgia, and multiple chemical sensitivity.[32] All of these diseases are marked by disputes over their "disease frames"—that is, the explanatory frameworks, schemas, and categories that we use to understand illness. The term "contested illness" is often used to describe these and other illnesses for which groups of laypeople, medical doctors, institutions, or organizations deny or question their existence. But contestations can spill over into controversies about other aspects of disease and illness. Doctors agree that autism and breast cancer exist, for example, but there is considerable contestation about these diagnoses' cause and treatment.[33]

Although doctors have long agreed that migraine exists, its severity and its social and cultural significance are contested. While people who have headache disorders often receive help for their symptoms, they are also likely to receive blame, be silenced, or be ignored. The discrepancy between the phenomenological experience of having migraine and the underwhelming response to this experience serves as a central puzzle guiding this book. How should we reconcile the fact that migraine is considered legitimate and serious in some circles, while ignored, dismissed, and delegitimated in others? This puzzle reveals the complexities inherent in the process of legitimating disease. I argue that migraine suffers from a "legitimacy deficit"—a phrase that highlights the complex, contingent, and contested character of legitimating disease. Legitimation is a process, not a status that is merely present or absent.

The concept of a legitimacy deficit represents a significant intervention into one of the principal lessons of social scientific research on health and illness: the extent to which mainstream medicine arbitrates what is a "real" and, therefore, a legitimate disease.[34] Common sense suggests that these distinctions should be based on biology. But, as many social scientists have demonstrated, disease categories reflect the specific historical and social contexts in which they are created. Disease entities are as social as they are biological. They form the basis for individual and collective identities, guide public policy, structure bureaucratic institution building, and organize clinical encounters.[35] Moreover, disease frames are transient, changing over time and across cultures. They are constantly being remade. Medical doctors change their mind about what is a disease as new knowledge is produced. As part of this process, doctors medicalize some conditions, like pregnancy or addiction. More rarely, doctors reject other conditions, like homosexuality, as medical states all together. Biology is only one of the factors that play a role in guiding these choices. Social, cultural, and historical forces also shape disease categories and explanatory models.[36] As a result, our categories of disease are never simply objective scientific stories about the body; they are stories about the culture in which they are created.

Sociologists have typically defined legitimacy "as a state of appropriateness ascribed to an actor, object, system, structure, process, or action resulting from its integration with institutionalized norms, values, and beliefs."[37] Theorists writing about the social construction of illness have argued that legitimacy in medicine is primarily dictated by a reductionist epistemology—that is, in Western societies, diseases are legitimate when real, and "real" refers to symptoms that can be linked to an identifiable, biological pathology.[38] Ideally, the pathology should be "specific," meaning that the pathology ought to uniformly produce a typical outcome in any man or woman no matter what his or her setting. In this reductionist view, which is based on germ theory, diseases are able to exist outside of individuals, independent of their manifestation in any particular person, and abstracted from social environments.

A range of proxies may serve as evidence of an underlying dysfunction in cases where a known, specific pathology has yet to be discovered. First, an association with a known pathogen can help legitimate a disease. For example, historian Robert Aronowitz points out that, early in its history, people believed that chronic fatigue syndrome might have a relationship with Epstein-Barr virus. This potential relationship made chronic fatigue syndrome more credible, thus attracting attention from clinicians and researchers.[39] The invention of effective pharmaceuticals is a second way to legitimate disorders. For example, in a classic article, sociologist Peter Conrad argues that the widespread use of Ritalin for the treatment of hyperactivity in children facilitated the creation of the diagnosis "hyperkinesis" (eventually known as attention deficit disorder), even though a causal mechanism had yet to be discovered.[40] Third, a somatic basis for disease can sometimes be inferred from sophisticated brain-imaging technologies, such as MRIs and PET scans, that show a difference between "normal" and sick brains. These images can be read to imply that otherwise invisible disorders, like depression, schizophrenia, and chronic pain, reside in the brain, thus creating the sense that these disorders are real.[41] Advocates may also attempt to legitimate illnesses by arguing that, no matter what their cause, illnesses produce huge economic and public health burdens.[42] In this case, ontology is grounded in an economic, rather than a biological, reality.

Medicalization theorists often maintain that the creation of a diagnosis (or "naming and framing") is crucially important in the process of transforming a set of symptoms into a legitimate disease. Certainly, diagnosis is an important tool for patients and physicians, who must use it to navigate the bureaucracies that govern health and illness in the United States.[43] In addition, beyond providing access to care and services, diagnosis plays an important cultural role in legitimating the experience of being ill for people who feel sick. The mere act of a doctor giving an illness a name can make a patient feel as if his or her experience has been acknowledged and accepted.[44] But while diagnosis (as well as effective drugs, imaging technologies, and economic reports) can be useful in establishing legitimacy, scholars generally believe the social legitimacy granted by it to be weaker than that offered by the presence of specific biological mechanisms.

Migraine complicates the relationship between specific disease and legitimation. Migraine has a well-established diagnosis, a subspecialty in medicine that is devoted to its treatment, brain imaging that illustrates a migraine in process, pharmacological interventions, research that links certain forms of migraine to genetic mutations, insurance companies and policy makers that recognize its existence (albeit to a limited degree), and a pharmaceutical industry that already markets some drugs to treat it and which is trying to develop more. And while researchers have not yet articulated a specific cause of migraine, they have developed a neurobiological model to explain much of the migraine process. Moreover, migraine differs from most of the contested illnesses that have been studied in that it has been defined as a medical diagnosis for hundreds, if not thousands, of years. Yet these advances have so far not been sufficient to validate the experiences of those with migraine, nor to bring resources to the study and treatment of migraine.

Legitimation, therefore, must depend on something more than the discovery of biomedical pathology. Legitimation also has a moral dimension. In other words, for a disease to be fully legitimated, the people who have it must be viewed as deserving of care and resources. Symptoms are never just reported—they are reported from particular people, who may belong to social groups that are more or less likely to be believed. Likewise, the public perception of a disease—and its relative importance—may hinge on the stereotypes of the social group with which it is associated. This aspect of legitimation is closely linked to stigma, which refers to a set of socially and culturally embedded prejudicial attitudes that discredit, taint, and devalue individuals.[45]

The relationship between legitimacy and stigma is particularly clear in diseases that are biomental.[46] Cultures that still implicitly assume that "body" is "real" and "mind" is "unreal" threaten the legitimacy of illnesses by casting doubt on the moral integrity of an ill person. A person complaining of ambiguous symptoms puts his or her credibility on the line. In the absence of an objective test that can prove the existence of a disease, the onus is on the individual to find a way to be rescued from any taint of malingering. I mean malingering here not in its narrow usage, which is limited to the exaggeration or feigning of illness, but in a broader sense suggested by its etymology, which comes from the French word *malingre*, a word formed from the prefix *mal*—"wrongly, improperly"—plus *haingre*—"weak." That is, malingering extends not just to the person who is consciously faking his or her symptoms, but to the person who ought to be fine, but is in some way "improperly weak." The malingerer, therefore, includes those who are disabled by the kinds of everyday ailments that the rest of us seem to cope with on a regular basis. We have idioms to describe this kind of person: they "make a mountain out of a molehill," and "cry wolf" at every ache and pain. In some contexts, like the emergency room, they may be characterized as drug seekers, complaining just so they can receive narcotics. Blacks and poor people may be more susceptible to such accusations than whites and the middle class. In other contexts, like work or the doctor's office, people with invisible symptoms may be characterized by feminized descriptors: neurotic, hypochondriacal, or sensitive. Women may be more prone to such labels than men, who are more likely to be perceived as stoic.

We can see this gender bias at work in the clinic, where it has been alleged that physicians prescribe less pain medication for women than they do for men, even though women experience more pain than men.[47] While little work of this nature has been done with migraine, one small study has shown that women are more likely than men to be diagnosed with migraine, yet once diagnosed, they are more likely than men to be prescribed antidepressants and tranquilizers, rather than pain medication.[48] Some researchers suggest that women receive less pain medication because they tend to be viewed as overly emotional, or even hysterical. Certainly, physicians routinely blame emotional factors for women's pain, whereas men's pain is more frequently attributed to bodily causes.[49] Less clear, but no less relevant, is how these and other stereotypes about moral character shape the relationship between race, class, pain, and perception.

If the first component of legitimacy is epistemological (how do we know that the disease is real?) and the second is moral (are people sick with this disease deserving of help?), then the third component of legitimacy is institutional. The Latin root of legitimacy, *lex*, means "law," suggesting that there is a political element to determining which entities are worthy of attention and resources. Indeed, sociologists typically use legitimacy to capture a generally held belief that an institution, a problem, or a leader is just and valid. In other words, legitimacy also refers to the ways in which institutional attention and other resources are allocated to the treatment of various diagnoses. Resources, in this sense, is a broad umbrella term that can include everything from the amount of federal funding allocated to the study of disease, to media attention, to the time that physicians spend learning about and treating a particular disease, to the number of sick days that employers are willing to grant to workers. There is a multidirectional relationship between legitimacy and resources—fully legitimate diseases receive more resources. However, as historian Keith Wailoo has demonstrated in the case of sickle cell anemia, diseases can also owe their legitimation to institutional logics—little attention was paid to sickle cell anemia or its sufferers until it became a model disease for new research agendas focused on molecular biology.[50]

Understanding the cultural politics of headache disorders therefore requires not only an account of how politics shape cultural meanings about what is real, true, and authentic, but also an examination of how cultural meanings affect headache disorders' fortunes in the political economy of disease, in which diseases compete with each other for resources. This analysis is crucial, especially given recent research demonstrating that policy makers disseminate research funds partly in response to the perceived worthiness of the patient population to be helped.[51] Resources will falter if a patient population is understood as weak, sensitive, demanding, or malingering. In contrast, patient populations that are understood in positive terms have an advantage when competing for limited funds. At the same time, it also must be recognized that a legitimacy deficit can be reduced via the allocation of resources, even in the absence of other markers that a collection of symptoms are real. For example, federal research funds can attract physicians and researchers to study a set of symptoms before a specific disease mechanism has been identified. Thus, for a diagnosis to achieve full legitimacy, it must have more than just a specific disease mechanism; patients who have the diagnosis must be constructed as deserving of care and resources, and those resources must be made available to them.

Gendering Specific Disease

Migraine stakeholders promote the neurobiological paradigm for headache disorders because they assume that explanations that invoke the brain transcend problems of moral character. But this is asking too much of somatic explanations. As many feminist science studies scholars have argued, explanatory frameworks are never value-neutral descriptions of what is going on in the body. Indeed, the most potent stories that knowledge about the body tells have to do with social hierarchies involving gender, race, and class.[52]

Feminist scholars have long noted that women's bodies are considered deviant, even when they behave in completely normal ways. For example, biomedicine treats pregnancy and menopause as diseases, even though both of these bodily states are normal and even desired for women.[53] Scholars have also uncovered that gender organizes how we understand the body, even when body parts are not directly related to biological sex. Anthropologist Emily Martin provides a classic example of this phenomenon at work in textbook representations of the immune system.[54] T cells, she argues, are often depicted as masculine leaders, who order subservient, feminized B cells to do the work of the immune system. Other scholars have discovered that the gendered subtext of disease is resilient and can persist, even as explanatory frameworks shift. For example, even though the invention of Prozac radically changed how doctors and the public think of mental illness, gender remains a salient feature in representations of depression.[55]

These insights from feminist research can help explain why a neurobiological model may be insufficient to legitimate migraine. Although neurobiology offers a biological explanation for migraine, this explanatory framework may have less power to legitimate migraine if it is understood in terms that replicate already existing assumptions about men and women in pain. At first blush, it can be difficult to understand how the body parts and processes involved in migraine, like the brain and neurotransmitters, might be gendered. (That biomedicine views the body as ahistorical and not amenable to cultural analysis makes gendering even more difficult to see.)[56] But through ethnographic observation, close readings of medical texts, and a comparative analysis between migraine and cluster headache, demonstrate that the neurobiological paradigm reproduces gendered notions of how men and women experience pain by ascribing moral characteristics to biological processes.

Gendering, in this context, refers to the way a person, object, subject, image, symbol, or metaphor is positioned within a gender system, which is a system of arbitrary hierarchies (e.g., across race, class, religion, sexual orientation, etc.) that have become ingrained in our cultural and institutional lives. These hierarchies are structured by binary oppositions, which ultimately justify unequal power relations.[57] We distinguish, for example, between nature/nurture, master/slave, thought/feeling, aggression/passivity, public/private, logic/intuition, rationality/emotion, and ultimately, man/woman. In each case, the first term of the "opposites" is associated with males, and the second with females. Likewise, society values the first set of terms over the second. By positioning discourses between these binary oppositions, gender signifies relationships of power.[58]

These dichotomies may encode meanings that have nothing to do with male or female bodies, specifically. That is, when an object or a cultural representation aligns with one side of a dichotomy, it becomes tied to that gender, even when a body is absent. For example, a minivan is discursively linked to children, groceries, and families in a way that is immediately recognizable as feminine. In contrast, an SUV may serve the same practical purpose, but is represented with the more masculine (or, at least, androgynous) concepts of the outdoors, sports, and adventure. Little qualitative difference may exist between how minivans and SUVs are used, but we make sense of them within a gendered discourse.

Gender as a signifier is not fixed to its meaning. In other words, very few men and women actually fit into all of their stereotyped values. Gender transgression happens all the time and may be more or less accepted in different contexts. Nevertheless, these dichotomies serve as a template for how we understand diseases and illness behavior. In this book, I illustrate this phenomenon by contrasting migraine, which is typically associated with women, with cluster headache, which is typically associated with men. I argue that it is meaningful that people who have migraine and cluster headache are constructed as having brains that operate in highly gendered ways: migraine affects a feminized, sensitive nervous system, which demands too much of its surroundings, while the brain of a cluster headache patient is constructed in masculine terms—hyperrational, but prone to risk taking.

Feminist theory can help us understand why it is that migraine passes some thresholds for legitimacy (in that it is fully medicalized) but remains woefully undertreated, underfunded, and under-resourced. By taking into account the gendering of neurobiological explanations, we can understand how people with migraine continue to be understood as weak, whiny hypochondriacs who cannot tolerate the aches and pains that come with everyday life, even as they are framed as having a brain disease. Thus, the legitimacy deficit persists in culture, in the clinic, and in policy circles.

A Science Studies Approach

To understand this legitimacy deficit, I followed the idea of headache through various cultural discourses.[59] This multisited ethnography allowed me to see how the perceived ordinariness of head pain wove itself into the rhetoric and practices of stakeholders in headache medicine, including headache specialists, pharmaceutical advertisers, and advocates. I took a science studies approach, examining each stakeholder as a knowledge producer with a perspective firmly situated in a cultural, economic, and political context. I also recognized that these groups would likely be deeply involved in the contests surrounding migraine's legitimacy. Based on feminist science studies literature, I hypothesized that gender would play an important role in how headache disorders are understood, but I wasn't sure how it would matter or if gender could alter how much legitimacy an invisible, chronic pain condition received. To find out, my analysis includes a comparative case study examining migraine, a diagnosis thought to be more prevalent among women than men, next to cluster headache, a diagnosis with a male-dominated demographic profile.

My work began at professional headache conferences where doctors and advocates meet to present and discuss the latest research in headache medicine. Over the years, I attended ten of these, using them as opportunities to listen to talks, view research posters, participate in pharmaceutical-sponsored events, chat with participants and organizers, and interview twenty-five of the top headache specialists in the United States about their work and their visions for the future of headache medicine. I supplemented these observations with targeted literature reviews of contemporary headache research. I also wanted to know where these ideas came from, so I historicized contemporary headache medicine with archival research extending back to the nineteenth century.

My research followed headache into private industry. I first encountered pharmaceutical companies at headache conferences, where they advertised their products to specialists and networked with doctors. Through ethnographic observation, content analysis of direct-to-consumer advertising, and interviews with two marketing executives, I witnessed and documented the various ways in which headache medicine and the pharmaceutical industry are intermeshed.

I also followed the work of headache advocates, many of whom have allied with headache specialists to change the way that migraine is understood. This fieldwork started in Italy in 2003, where I met with the World Headache Alliance (WHA) and their members. The WHA is an umbrella group that unites headache advocates around the world. On the same trip, I also met cluster headache advocates, who had traveled to Italy to attend a "Cluster Club" meeting. Soon after, new advocacy efforts located in America began to pop up. I followed these efforts with great interest, including the newly formed Alliance for Headache Disorders Advocacy (AHDA), which lobbies Congress to increase funding for research on headache disorders. I attended four of their "Headache on the Hill" events and participated in their lobbying efforts.

These efforts, however, were organized by physicians, rather than patients. Grassroots activities were, by and large, restricted to the Internet, which had become an increasingly exciting place for migraine advocacy from 2004 onward. I began my research into these online communities by conducting formal interviews with fourteen headache advocates, some of whom run formal organizations (recognized as such by tax status), but most of whom acted alone, either as bloggers or as authors. I also conducted a content analysis of twenty-one migraine and cluster headache blogs, as well as an analysis of discussions that happened in migraine and cluster headache discussion forums.

This research resulted in a thick description of the politics involved in the construction of headache disorders. In the end, I argue that stakeholders' best attempts to legitimate migraine are undermined by cultural meanings of headache and migraine that are overlaid with assumptions about gender. These gender assumptions overdetermine how medical knowledge about headache disorders is produced, disseminated, and used.

A Cultural Approach

I paid particular attention to culture, believing that it is culture that ultimately shapes how knowledge is produced, by making some ideas natural and others unthinkable. Here, I draw on Ann Swidler's conception of culture as a toolkit filled with stories, symbols, rituals, and worldviews that people use in varying configurations to solve problems.[60] These cultural notions often appear as common sense, which makes them all the more potent.

To this end, I titled this book *Not Tonight* to call upon Freud's reminder that jokes summon explosive realities that people would prefer not to

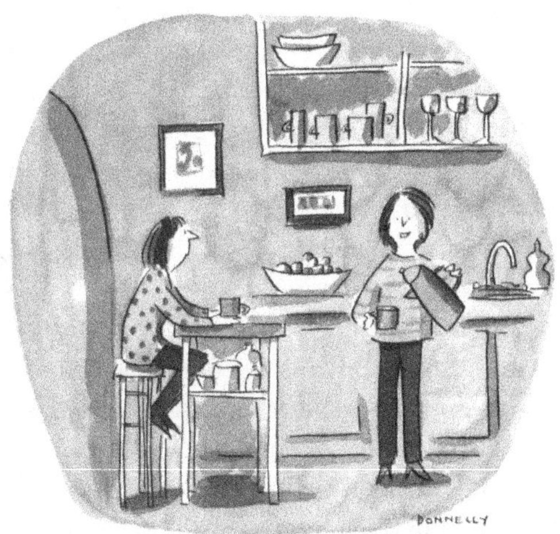

FIGURE I.2 One woman to another as they are about to have coffee. "I had a headache, too, but he went away." Issue publication date 03/24/1997. Liza Donnelly / The New Yorker Collection / www.cartoonbank.com.

think about in ordinary conversation. It is an interesting and important cultural fact that *Roget's Thesaurus* lists "spouse" and "wife" as synonyms for headache. In other contexts, "headache" immediately suggests a series of misogynist jokes:[61] "One of the side effects of Viagra is a headache. Every time I take a pill, my wife gets a headache!" Or a cartoon depicting a woman entering the bedroom with a baseball bat who says to the man in bed "I don't feel like having sex. But tonight, I won't be the one having the headache!" One of my favorites is a *New Yorker* cartoon with two women sitting casually in a kitchen, chatting over a cup of coffee. The caption, which reads "I had a headache, too, but he went away," is funny because it puns on the three most common headache metaphors—headache as an excuse for women to avoid sex, headaches as a result of stress, and headache as a synonym for a significant other. It is assumed that the audience will be familiar enough with these multiple meanings of headache that are layered and played against each other to pick up the joke (see figure I.2).

"The power of a metaphor," wrote Clifford Geertz, "derives precisely from the interplay between the discordant meanings it symbolically coerces into a unitary conceptual framework and from the degree to which that coercion is successful in overcoming the psychic resistance such semantic tension inevitably generates in anyone in a position to perceive it."[62] Repeated use of metaphors and imagery—for example, headaches and avoidance of sex or headaches and weakness—eventually connects these two otherwise disparate ideas. Once these metaphors become commonplace, they have the power to define the "really real" for people. What begins as a literary or visual comparison results in a powerful version of reality. Eventually, this connection is so naturalized that it appears as plain and easy as common sense.

Interestingly, the clichés about women, sex, and migraine are so widespread that they have generated both scientific and cultural inquiries into whether migraine is, in fact, a common excuse for avoiding sex. James Couch, a neurologist and headache specialist, conducted the most famous of these studies and concluded that people with migraine counterintuitively use sex to halt a migraine in process. Two-thirds of the women he surveyed said that sex was an effective means of reducing head pain and a third claimed that sex could abort their pain altogether.[63] The media usually pick up these sorts of studies with headlines like "Headaches: 'Yes Tonight, Dear.'" These findings are also popular fodder in sex-advice columns, leading to the publication of sex columns like this one written by Yvonne Kristín Fulbright in *Fox News Health* blogs: A reader asks "[Can] sex also act as a type of headache medicine? I want something to say the next time my wife tells me she's not in the mood because she has a 'headache.'" Fulbright's answer was not a sensitive intervention into this man's presumptions about his wife's motives, but instead a simple yes. She cites in her answer a study in which undergraduate students reported that "headache" was a primary motivation for having sex.[64] That these studies are done at all is testament to the power of the "not tonight" cliché—one would not expect that a person with a knife wound or in the midst of say, a seizure, would want to engage in sex either. But no study need investigate whether this is indeed true. (Incidentally, there does exist a variety of headache that is triggered by orgasm. "Primary headache associated with sexual activity"—or what was previously known as "coital cephalalgia"—is an unusual disorder characterized by severe head pain that occurs suddenly, often near the time of orgasm, and which lasts for up to twenty-four hours.

Culture works by making some ideas natural and others unthinkable. This book casts a new light on how, exactly, our shared schemas and beliefs are related to the process of disease legitimization and social problem formation. Chances are that we all know someone who has a headache disorder. So why do headache disorders continue to be neglected? And what does their neglect say about the political and cultural processes structuring the creation of knowledge and health policy about pain? Understanding this process requires a fundamental understanding that disease is more than an objective biological phenomenon—it is a source of rich cultural meaning.

Plan of the Book

In chapter 1, I provide a historical overview of the shifting biomedical understanding of migraine over the past three hundred years. This overview allows me to track the origin of migraine's association with weak, gendered personalities. My history starts in the eighteenth century when doctors began theorizing a relationship between illness, nerves, and sensibility. I then follow shifting understandings of the mind-body relationship in migraine, from nineteenth-century formulations of migraine as a disorder of upper-class intellectual men and hysterical women, to the influential concept of "migraine personality" in the 1940s in which women with migraine were described as uptight neurotics who withheld sex, to contemporary discussions of people with migraine as experiencing high rates of comorbidity with the highly gendered diagnoses of depression and anxiety.

Although the framework for understanding migraine shifts considerably across time, I argue that, throughout, medical doctors make presumptions about the *kind* of person who gets migraine. In each era, this person has a particular set of moral characteristics, which are both highly gendered and which help guide how the person with migraine is treated more generally. This history holds important lessons about the relationship between medicine, culture, science, ideology, illness, and meaning.

In chapter 2, I analyze the notion that migraine has recently undergone a paradigm shift—an idea that permeates headache specialists' narrative retellings of their discipline's own history. Headache specialists describe migraine as having undergone a revolutionary transformation from a condition "once believed to be a disorder of neurotic women," but which is now understood as a "neurobiological disease." Headache specialists are excited about this transformation, in large part because it allows them to leave behind a history that in many ways appears to be nonscientific, if not completely sexist. I argue, however, that this paradigmatic shift is driven, in part, by a professional desire to build a more credible and legitimate profession. Nevertheless, this move toward the brain has failed to degender migraine and instead has created a new, highly gendered "kind" of migraine patient—a person in possession of a hypersensitive, demanding "migraine brain." I argue that the migraine brain is not much different than the psychosomatic migraine patient that it has replaced, and, in fact, that it reifies many of the gendered assumptions that psychosomatic medicine made.

Chapter 3 turns its attention toward an online embodied health movement aimed at changing how people perceive migraine. Within a culture that diminishes pain, people with migraine report that the legitimacy deficit fundamentally shapes not only their experience but also their self-concept. Some groups of people with migraine, collectively gathered in online communities, have sought refuge in the neurobiological paradigm—a model of migraine that they view not only as best able to represent their embodied experience, but as the best way of representing migraine politically. Although their narratives of delegitimation are highly gendered, they are seemingly unbothered by the gendered characterization of the migraine brain that they have embraced.

Chapter 4 takes a closer look at the explicit marketing strategies used by the pharmaceutical industry to sell migraine drugs. The information, tactics, metaphors, catchphrases, and images communicated via promotional schemes not only increase the visibility of those conditions for which drugs are advertised, they also inject public discourse with a new set of meanings and symbols with which to understand migraine. While in some ways new pharmaceutical technologies have facilitated biological explanations for migraine that have moved the discourse away from "neurotic females," the analysis in this chapter suggests that many so-called outdated cultural assumptions about migraine—as an unimportant condition that only affects a particular kind of woman—remain embedded in the patchwork of images, narratives, and rhetoric produced by the pharmaceutical industry.

Chapter 5 draws on an in-depth case study of cluster headache to ask what headache medicine might look like if migraines were male. Cluster headache is a rare form of headache that is notoriously painful and dramatic. Cluster headache is also unusual because, unlike other pain disorders, which tend to affect women, cluster headache is thought to predominantly affect men. In contrast to migraine, cluster headache researchers rarely, if ever, discuss problems related to the status and legitimacy of the condition. Rather, they point to the severity of cluster headache's symptoms, which are framed as uniquely masculine, so much so that they bring "even the strongest of men to their knees." This masculine discourse even extends to female cluster headache patients, who are recast as women who lack feminine qualities or whose bodies are punishing them for transgressing traditional gender roles. This physical and psychological description of cluster headache (aka the cluster profile) has been remarkably resilient, even as more recent studies undermine these findings. On the other hand, people with cluster headache are very concerned with legitimacy, describing how they appear "wimpy" when people confuse "cluster headache" with "headache" or "migraine." The overt masculinity embedded in cluster headache medicine makes clear how cultural assumptions of gender influence migraine medicine and how gender shapes the experience of headache disorders.

So why has the brain done so little to change cultural meanings of headache disorders? In the conclusion, I argue that biomedicalization has not been enough to legitimate migraine, since—even as a "brain disease"—migraine remains plagued by gendered images, metaphors, and stereotypes. This analysis of headache disorders not only provides an important vantage point for understanding how cultural beliefs about the relationship between gender, class, and pain are inscribed and reinscribed into bodies, it also demonstrates how these factors shape the credibility of people in pain.

CHAPTER ONE

All in Her Mind

Migraine blurs the boundaries between mind and body in complicated ways. Take the story of Civil War Union general Ulysses S. Grant. On the evening of April 8, 1865, Grant's army had finally cornered Robert E. Lee's now exhausted Confederate army in Appomattox, Virginia. But Grant felt terrible. General Lee refused to surrender, and Grant was suffering from a severe "sick headache"—a condition that shares much in common with today's migraine.

Grant got little rest as the armies settled down for the night. "I spent the night," he wrote, "in bathing my feet in hot water and mustard, and putting mustard plasters on my wrists and the back part of my neck, hoping to be cured by morning." Grant felt much the same the next day until he received a letter with better news: Lee had changed his mind. "When the officer reached me, I was still suffering from the sick headache; but the instant I saw the contents of the note I was cured." With his headache gone, Grant met with Lee and negotiated a peace that would end the bloody war.[1]

Grant's vanishing headache dramatically illustrates the complicated interrelationship between mind and body in headache disorders. Anxiety or stress might exacerbate an underlying tendency to get migraine, but then, as in Grant's experience, a turn of mood can abort even the worst attack. In contrast, for many people, migraine only comes during moments of relaxation. (Doctors used to call this phenomenon "weekend headaches" or "let-down migraines.")[2] Or migraines stay away during extreme stress, only to return in response to everyday aggravations. Joan Didion tries to explain these contradictions in her own migraines: "Tell me that my house is burned down, my husband has left me, that there is gunfighting in the streets and panic in the banks, and I will not respond by getting a headache. It comes instead when I am fighting not an open but a guerrilla war with my own life, during weeks of small household confusions, lost laundry, unhappy help, canceled appointments, on days when the telephone rings too much and I get no work done and the wind is coming up. On days like that my friend comes uninvited."[3]

The odd relationship between emotions and the onset and frequency of migraine is just one facet of how mind and body interact in migraine. The very experience of migraine can sometimes feel like a voyage to the fringes of the mental. This is especially true of migraine aura, which brings with it a diverse set of symptoms, some of which are surreal (hallucinations of sight, sound, and smell) and some of which are affective (elation, irritability, anxiety, or overactivity).[4] Novelist Siri Hustvedt describes her auras as a "lunatic borderland" that provide pleasure, inspiration, and entertainment.[5] Neurologist Oliver Sacks has mused that the fortification patterns he sees during visual aura might connect him to universal archetypes of human experience, noting that these patterns are the same as those used in the Alhambra, Zapotec architecture, bark paintings of Australian Aboriginal artists, and Swazi basketry.[6] He suggests that the universality of these patterns might be rooted in the neuronal structure of humanity's shared visual cortex, but the reader can't miss the spiritual subtext of his essay. Lewis Carroll, on the other hand, envisions aura as magical and horrible. People in the headache community often say that his masterpiece, *Alice in Wonderland*, was inspired by his own experience with migraine aura. Some people with migraine, for example, experience the sensation of having body parts much larger or smaller than they actually are. Alice frequently feels the same way. After drinking the contents of a strange bottle, she says: "I must be shutting up like a telescope. And so it was indeed: She was now only 10 inches high."[7]

Not everyone finds these perceptual shifts as preternaturally romantic as Sacks, Hustvedt, and Carroll. An intense feeling of dread can also precede migraine attacks. Not infrequently, people with migraine lose fundamental language skills just prior to or during an attack. And treatment can complicate matters, as many medications used in the prevention and treatment of migraine have cognitive side effects including depression, difficulty concentrating, and forgetting words.

These examples demonstrate why Oliver Sacks has argued that

migraine ought to be seen as a prime example of the "absolute continuity of mind and body."[8] Over the centuries, physicians have placed migraine in various positions along the mind/body spectrum.[9] Headache experts currently consider migraine a somatic disorder rooted in the brain. But this is a break from the past. Up until thirty years ago, doctors primarily viewed migraine as having both a psychological and a somatic basis. In what follows, I trace these historical understandings of migraine from the nineteenth-century understanding of migraine as a disorder of upper-class intellectuals, to the influential concept of the "migraine personality" in mid-twentieth-century America, and finally to contemporary theories of comorbidity.

Each of these formulations describes the person with migraine as having particular qualities—that is, a distinctive moral character. And since moral descriptors tend to have gendered components, so do historical explanations of migraine. Of course, it is fair to say that any historical narrative of medicine will dredge up discourses that sound explicitly sexist by today's standards. As cultural theorist Paula Treichler points out, analyses that accuse medicine of sexism tell us little that we don't already know. Instead, she recommends analyses that interrogate how these representations of disease are "produced, disseminated, understood, and put to use" because they can help us contextualize how contemporary frameworks for understanding headache disorders continue to perpetuate stereotypical ideas about gender.[10] In the account that follows, I pay close attention to how, at each historical turn, biomedical discourses come to enact and reinforce cultural narratives about gender, class, and pain via the encoded inclusion of moral character. After all, the credibility and the legitimacy of a disorder—and how much we, as a society, choose to invest in its treatment—is intimately tied to how we perceive the moral character of the patient.

Victorians and the Nervous Temperament

In Western medicine, headache disorders have long been understood as complaints that are rooted in the body but that maintain intimate relationships with emotions.[11] Even as far back as Plato's *Charmides*, Socrates refuses to give the hero headache medicine till first he had eased his troubled mind; body and soul, he said, must be cured together, as head and eyes.[12] Galen, whose theory of "hemicrania" dominated medicine until the seventeenth century, speculated "certain natures . . . may end up suffering from headache if they lead an intemperate life."[13]

This association between headache and emotions persisted even as more modern physicians began to favor biological explanations of head pain. In the late seventeenth century, Thomas Willis (1621–1675), the "father of modern neurology," wrote about migraine as a "nervous" disorder, locating the pain in the physiological structures of the brain. Yet despite this fundamental shift in how migraine physiology was understood, Willis warned that treatment of migraine in a patient would be "more difficult, if hypochondriacal, or hysterick."[14] Samuel Tissot's (1728–1797) highly influential eighteenth-century treatise on migraine attributed the disorder to disturbed function of the stomach, but argued that this disturbance could be created by emotional and intellectual factors:[15] James Mease (1771–1846), writing in 1832, agreed that the stomach was fundamental to understanding the disorder, but cautioned, "The passions of the mind must be kept under with especial care. Every mental irritation will add strength to the disease, and retard the wholesome operation of the remedies prescribed for its cure."[16]

References to mind and body, like the ones made by Willis, Tissot and Mease, were common in eighteenth- and nineteenth-century medicine. Victorian doctors, especially, made few distinctions between mind and body; it was simply assumed that emotions, mental impatience, lifestyle, and passions could affect, and even bring on, all sorts of disease. Because distinctions between mind and body were so rarely made, all of nineteenth-century medicine could profitably be described as psychosomatic.[17]

The late nineteenth century witnessed the development of increasingly sophisticated theories about the physiological mechanisms of migraine. Physicians began to debate whether migraine should be attributed to disruptions in the nervous system or to dilation and constriction of the cranial vessels. But they agreed on one thing: the person with migraine had a "nervous temperament" that lent him an unusual intelligence, an active imagination, and a susceptibility to illness. This sensitive nervous structure produced a moral character that could be inherited from one's family or cultivated through intense study. Nevertheless, the temperament was understood as an organic (somatic) phenomenon. How might this work?

Physician John Symonds (1807–1881) laid out a new framework for how a nervous temperament could exacerbate physical ills. "Say that a wasp has stung the dorsum of the foot," explained Symonds in an 1848 lecture on migraine. "The pain may soon extend to the whole foot, or even the whole limb, without any corresponding extension of the local irritation caused by the wasp poison."[18] His point being that, in a normal person, pain can and does travel "sympathetically" away from its original source. But the nervous system of a "nervous" person is organized differently: "In different subjects there is a vast difference in the readiness with which these communications are made. Persons are called irritable, nervous, susceptible, hysterical, when the proclivities to such communication is very marked."[19] The nervous temperament, Symonds continued, did not affect all sectors of society equally. Rather, it tended to afflict "persons of very lively emotions and delicate sensitivity, easily perturbed mind, easily put off their sleep, [and] those who have the aesthetical and imaginative elements highly developed. It is also the frequent accompaniment and curse of high intellectual endowments."[20]

Symonds was repeating an old and well-accepted theory of nervous disease that had circulated for over one hundred years.[21] In 1733, George Cheyne (1671–1743), a fashionable Scottish doctor in London at the time, wrote a widely read book, *The English Malady*, that explained poor health via degradation of the nervous system. Nerve strength guaranteed health. Nerves that were "too lax, feeble and unelastik" bred pathology and made one susceptible to environmental changes.[22] For example, people with weak nerves felt "too much Pain and Uneasiness from cold or frosty Weather" and "too great a Degree of Sensibility or Easiness of being acted upon by external objects."[23] He blamed a combination of a heavy, unhealthy English diet; sedentary professions; and the hectic, noisy, and polluted London lifestyle for further burdening the weak nervous system.

Cheyne did not, however, see weak nerves as entirely unhealthy. The thinner and more fragile the nerve, the more quickly it could transmit a quality called "sense." "Sensibility" conveyed aesthetic, intellectual, and social refinement, made one a "quick Thinker," and provided the "most lively imagination." Talented people were born with "organs finer, quicker, more agile, and sensible, and perhaps more numerous than others."[24] In contrast, "*brute* Animals have few or none, at least none that belong to *Reflection*; Vegetables certainly none at all."[25] Sensibility could be cultivated, but was also seen to be biologically rooted and inborn, determined directly by the exquisiteness and delicacy of one's nerves. It was simply an unfortunate irony that refinement of nerves coupled so tightly with susceptibility to illness. People of good breeding, high sensibility, and excellent moral character were expected to come down with nervous disorders, like hysteria, hypochondria, or the "Vapours."[26]

Cheyne's description of the nervous system and its disorders mirrored the clearly demarcated race and class boundaries of the time: the upper class with their weak nerves and sharp senses were biologically built for sedentary and intellectual professions, whereas the working class's (and African's) robust nerves and dull senses had the perfect build and aptitude for physical labor. But this logic presented a puzzle when it came to women, as they suffered from hysteria and other nervous disorders with greater frequency than men, but were not considered intellectually superior beings. Cheyne's contemporary, Bernard de Mandeville (1670–1733), laid out this problem in *A Treatise of the Hypochondriack and Hysterick Diseases*: "Studying and intense thinking are not to be alledg'd as a Cause in Women, whom we know (at least for the generality of them) to be so little guilty of it; and yet the Number of hysterick Women far exceeds that of hypochondriack Men."[27] The answer, Cheyne argued, lay in their "Deficiency of the Spirits." Women were simply born with weaker, finer, and more delicate nerves than men and, therefore, were not "made capable of running into the same Indiscretions or Excess of Sensual Pleasures" as were those born with "strong Fibres or Robust Constitutions."[28]

That women's "delicacy" (in personality, tastes, and sensibility) was the result of their "delicate" nervous systems became firmly entrenched in both scientific and popular imagination. This "nervous temperament" will be immediately familiar to those who have read eighteenth- and nineteenth-century novels, many of which valorized sensibility and the nervous temperament. For example, Jane Austen's Marianne Dashwood, the heroine in *Sense and Sensibility*, seeks a life filled with aesthetic pleasures and high culture.[29] It is no coincidence that she is also of delicate constitution, having nearly died after walking in a torrential downpour. Her sensitive nervous system allows for superior tastes and intellect, but leaves her flailing with a weak constitution.

John Symonds's 1848 lecture about the relationship between migraine and nervous temperament shared these gender and class assumptions. But he added a new dimension: "Such persons may also feel pains which have taken their origin from mere ideas."[30] And, thus, Symonds became the first—but certainly not the last—headache doctor to suggest in print that head pain might be caused entirely by suggestion. Or to phrase his contribution more accurately, suggestion could only bring on disease in a person whose body had already been weakened by "nervous temperament."[31]

The Lingering Nervous Temperament

Not long after Symonds's lecture, two competing theories of the biological basis of migraine emerged, each with long-lasting consequences. Both theories identified migraine as biological, albeit positing different underlying mechanisms. Despite their biological orientation, however, both theories made ample use of highly gendered assumptions related to moral character. The nervous temperament remained a salient feature of migraine in the late nineteenth century.

The first theory posited that symptoms of migraine were due to vascular changes in cranial vessels. This was an ancient idea: physicians had implicated the vascular system in migraine since at least the seventeenth century. But in 1859, German physician Emil Du Bois Reymond (1818–1896) renewed these theories with his observation that his own face paled during migraine attacks—the cause, then, must be the vasoconstriction of cranial vessels.[32] In contrast, his compatriot, Möllendorf, noted in 1867, that his own face, as well as those of his patients, flushed during migraine attacks. Migraine, then, must be caused by either the expansion or dilation of cranial vessels. London medical lecturer Peter Wallwork Latham combined these two theories in 1873, arguing that Reymond and Möllendorf were both right. The migraine *began* with vasoconstriction, which would explain the visual and emotional symptoms preceding headache. But then the vasculature, exhausted by constriction, would over-dilate, causing the pain of migraine. He argued that his model could explain the varied expression of migraine symptoms:

> It is well known that the vision is disturbed by a diminished supply of blood to the brain—as, for instance, in the faintness, which is induced by haemorrhage. The patients become giddy; everything appears dark before them; perhaps they have, moreover, flashes of light before their eyes, or noises in their ears, and then become insensible, and sink to the ground. How often do we hear from persons who are dying from asthenia such expressions as the following? "How dark the room is; "I can't see"; "open the shutters"; telling us too plainly that the heart is powerless to drive the blood onward to the brain.[33]

Latham concludes that, during this process, "The vessels become distended, the head throbs and aches, and the pupil contracts."[34]

The second theory, which reemerged as an influential text in the late twentieth and early twenty-first centuries, was forwarded by English physician Edward Liveing (1832–1919) in 1873. Liveing, said to have migraine, proposed a neurogenic theory in a thick treatise published the same year as Latham's lectures. He argued that all headache disorders ought to be considered "megrim," and, furthermore, that they are a close relative of epilepsy. His rationale was that the central cause of megrim had to be "a primary and often hereditary vice or morbid disposition of the nervous system itself" caused by an "irregular accumulation and discharge of nerve force" that would trigger a "nerve storm."[35] (Neurologist John Hughlings Jackson, his contemporary, had offered this explanation for epilepsy.)[36] Liveing, moreover, rejected all vasomotor theories as inadequate to explain the myriad symptoms associated with megrim.

Contemporary neurologists consider Liveing's treaty to be the real nineteenth-century innovation in headache medicine,[37] but nineteenth-century physicians were dismissive. Latham, for example, was not at all happy with Liveing's assessment of megrim as a close cousin of epilepsy—a disorder that had the hereditary taint of criminals, prostitutes, psychopaths, and homosexuals. Latham was pleased that his vasomotor theory would free migraine of these unfortunate associations: "If we take this [a vasomotor] view of the disorder, you will perceive that it has (as was first suggested to me by my friend Dr. Edward Liveing) a relationship, though happily a very distant one, to epilepsy."[38]

Both Latham and Liveing draw on the notion of the nervous temperament to various degrees. Latham described people with migraine as "possess[ing] what is called the nervous temperament; their brains are very excitable, their senses acute, and their imaginations free."[39] Latham encoded this excitability into his vasomotor theory and descriptions of the migrainous body. People with migraine, he argued, had a vascular system that mirrored their mental exhaustion. It also reflected their overall physique, lending them "a general want of tone—a relaxed condition of the muscular and arterial systems . . . the pulse being rather small and soft, often decidedly slow, but much accelerated on slight exertion or excitement."[40] Tension and "over-work" could cause the vasculature to constrict. Once the tension passed, the vasculature was likely to dilate.[41]

Liveing's references to moral character were subtler. Liveing argued that megrim was transmitted via heredity, which linked megrim closely to epilepsy, insanity, and other nervous disorders. But heredity, alone, could not bring on megrim. One would only inherit a disposition. Megrim required an additional "influence or combination of circumstances to call it forth."[42] Liveing argued that a person must engage in a behavior to experience migraine; thus, he concluded, people who experienced migraine would cluster in certain professions because of the conditions of their work—they were likely to be "a literary man, a barrister, a member of parliament."[43] His argument was sociological. If "overworked students, literary men, artisans, and [seamstresses]" were more likely to get migraine, then "depressing influences of various kinds" were to blame. "The malady often disappears again when the causes which determined it are removed."[44]

From a contemporary perspective, one of the most striking features of nineteenth-century writings on headache disorders is the extent to which most authors presumed a masculine subject, writing about the implicit migraine patient as "he" and including case studies of male patients along with the women.[45] Nevertheless, most physicians understood migraine to affect more women than men, despite their references to barristers and members of Parliament. The extent to which this was true, however, was a point very much up for debate. In 1848, John Symonds reported the first quasi-systematic attempt to collect epidemiological data on migraine. His data, collected from hospital registrars and colleagues, found that seventy-six of ninety cases of "nervous headache" were female. "These numbers establish more strongly than I should have expected, the fact, which is testified by most of the old writers, that females are more frequent sufferers."[46] Liveing rejected Symonds's statistics, arguing that "to make it trustworthy it ought to be shown that the cases were drawn from a miscellaneous body of patients in which both sexes were fairly represented. It is highly improbable that this was the case."[47] Liveing agreed that women were more likely to be affected with megrim, but estimated that a more fair gender ratio would be five to four.

It is, however, difficult to tell exactly what these physicians were measuring. Each had his own classification system for headache disorders, and variations across these systems could significantly change any measurement of prevalence and the corresponding gender ratio. For example, while Liveing considered a wide range of symptoms to fall under the category "megrim," other physicians made distinctions between "neuralgic headaches," "hemicrania," "nervous headache," "clavus hystericus," and so forth. If women were systematically excluded from a single category like migraine, then epidemiological estimates of prevalence would include enormous variation. Substantial evidence suggests that, in fact, women who complained of headache were systematically given different diagnoses than men. *Clavus hystericus*, sometimes called "hysterical headache," is the clearest example of a gendered diagnostic category in this time period. In his *Treatises on the Diseases of the Nervous System*, James Ross describes hysterical headache as a variation of hysteria: "Hysterical Headache is met with in females, and is generally accompanied by other symptoms of hysteria. This form of headache is on the one hand closely allied to trigeminal neuralgia, and on the other to true migraine. The pain is sometimes diffused and deep-seated, but it is more frequently limited to one spot, and feels as if a nail were being driven through the skull; hence it is called 'clavus.' Hysterical headache is increased in severity during the menstrual period and by mental worry, whilst it is removed by amusement and anything which engages the attention."[48] "Hysterical tendencies" could distinguish the pain of clavus hystericus from other headache disorders, although authors were usually vague about what, exactly, constituted these symptoms. In his 1888 monograph on headache disorders, Allan Mclane Hamilton suggests only one objective distinction: "Hysterical women are very apt to complain of very great diffused hyperaesthesia of the scalp, so that the simple act of brushing the hair causes great distress."[49] (This complaint might now be diagnosed as allodynia, which is a pain condition associated with migraine.) Knowing which of his patients had what Hamilton called "neuralgia," which is described in his book as having a solid biological basis, and which were merely hysterical was important for treatment, as hysterics "are more apt than any others to form the opium habit, or that of alcoholism, and great care should be taken lest, by yielding to their demands, we foster something worse than the headache or hysteria."[50]

These arbitrary distinctions between nervous headache, neuralgias, and clavus hystericus in part reflected an evolution in how Victorians had begun to think about neuroses and the lines dividing mind and body. Traditionally, the nervous temperament and references to "nerves" more generally, did not, as we might think, automatically refer to psychological distress. Rather, these physicians were referring to a traditional and physicalist understanding of neurosis that had been handed down from the eighteenth century. Mental strain caused disease by way of weak and delicate nerves that became strained, stressed, and overstretched. But medical thinking on this topic was undergoing a massive upheaval during this time. Charles Darwin's theory of evolution had made heredity a popular way of thinking about nervous disease. Thinkers like Alexander Bain and Jean-Martin Charcot drew attention to the influence of the will over the body.

As a result, mid-nineteenth-century discourses on nervous disease were often contradictory and incoherent. A nervous temperament indicated a weak nervous system. But nervous systems could be weakened because of the strong emotions conjured up by weak temperaments. This irreducible circularity begged a question: which came first, psychopathology or heredity? Headache doctors in the twentieth century had answers.

The Rise of the Migraine Personality

The poles demarcating the mind/body continuum underwent significant shifts in the early twentieth century. On one end of the continuum, Sigmund Freud's highly influential writing on the unconscious mind emphasized the influence and power of the will over the body.[51] On the other end, a budding pharmaceutical industry was beginning to develop drugs that actually effected change in the body. At first glance, it might seem as if the latter of these two trends would have a more direct impact on the understanding and experience of headache disorders: the treatment of minor headaches improved dramatically with the discovery of aspirin in 1899.[52] In addition, physicians were discovering that ergotamine, a drug derived from rye, could terminate a migraine. That ergotamine was a known vasoconstrictor significantly strengthened Latham's vasomotor theory of migraine.[53] And, indeed, these pharmaceutical treatments did lead to new discoveries about the biological basis of migraine. But these discoveries came along around the same time that psychosomatic medicine was taking off as a medical specialty. As a result, new theories about the biological basis of migraine were accompanied by a new psychosomatic theory about the cause of migraine: the migraine personality.

It was Harold G. Wolff (1898–1962), the predominant headache researcher of the early twentieth century, who did the most to transform vasomotor and psychosomatic theories of migraine into scientific and popular gospel. Wolff, a neurologist at the New York Hospital–Cornell Medical Center, is often called the father of modern headache research.[54] He engaged in two long-lasting avenues of research from 1930 to his death in 1962. First, he demonstrated that cranial blood vessels were dilated during the headache that occurs when a person experiences a migraine; this work additionally provided much evidence supporting now-obsolete constriction theories of aura. Second, because Wolff viewed biology as responsive to the psyche, he pursued psychological explanations of migraine, popularizing psychosomatic theories of migraine, particularly the idea of a "migraine personality."

Wolff became interested in how blood vessels reacted during migraine while completing his neurological training with Stanley Cobb, a leading investigator into the biological roots of psychiatry at Harvard. After this training, Wolff traveled through Europe and Russia and studied with the most eminent scholars in the burgeoning field of psychoanalytic and behavioral research. His remarkable list of mentors include Otto Loewi, an Austrian winner of the Nobel Prize in physiology or medicine; Ivan Pavlov, the Russian psychologist who won a Nobel Prize in physiology or medicine for demonstrating how conditioning works in dogs; and Adolf Meyer, a Johns Hopkins psychiatrist who developed the notion of psychobiology. By the time he took his position at New York Hospital in 1932, Wolff had already been thinking about the defensive reaction patterns of individual behavior that could cause disease.[55] His interest was in moving beyond the typical Cartesian mind/body divide to understand how psyche, personality, and biology could simultaneously contribute to nervous disorders.

In particular, Wolff applied his broader hypotheses regarding the role of stress, personality, and behavior in disease to understanding vascular activity in migraine. Using simple materials, he set up rather ingenious experiments that allowed researchers to observe changes in the vascular structure of migraine subjects. Helen Goodell, Wolff's long-time assistant, provides a description of an early experiment, in which Wolff and his colleagues devised a tool that could measure the extent to which the vascular system dilated during migraine. Wolff induced migraine in subjects with intravenous injections of histamine. A needle and tabour were placed over the temporal artery and connected through a Rube Goldberg-esque mechanism that included an air system, mirrors, lights, and cameras. The result was an "old fashioned but ingenious way both intracranial and temporal artery pulsations could be recorded quite satisfactorily."[56]

Previous experiments had illustrated how histamine could instigate a throbbing headache, mimicking a migraine. These early experiments established that blood pressure dropped just after the injection and that the headache began as the blood pressure returned to normal. From these early results, researchers had already surmised that vasoconstriction was occurring somewhere in the vascular bed. But Wolff, with his clever new device, was able to obtain a *visible* measure of what was previously unseen. This objective evidence not only seemed to demonstrate that headache

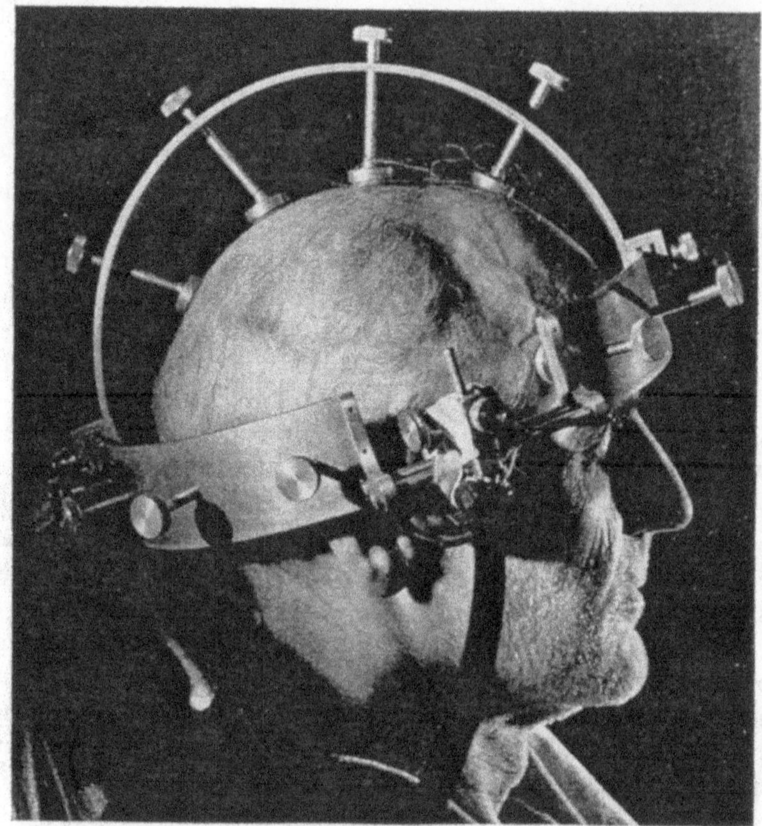

FIGURE 1.1 Wolff's experiment. Photograph by Fritz Goro, *Life* magazine.

began with vasodilation, but it demonstrated that this vasodilation was correlated to the amplitude of intracranial pulsations. In other words, the pulsing pain of migraine could be attributed to the vasodilation of cranial arteries. The thump, thump, thumping of the head had everything to do with the thump, thump, thumping of the heart. With time, Wolff's experiments became more technically sophisticated and brought him great fame and publicity (see figure 1.1).

In later experiments, Wolff tried to demonstrate that vasoconstriction early in a migraine attack caused migraine aura. In one such experiment, Wolff gave a small amount of amyl nitrate—a drug known to dilate blood vessels—to a medical student in the midst of an aura. The student's aura briefly disappeared. Later experiments demonstrated a similar effect when he administered carbon dioxide, another vasodilator, to research subjects with aura. These experiments were provocative, but Wolff viewed them as speculative. Nevertheless, his colleagues in medicine readily adopted his findings as fact.

Wolff's objective measures of migraine physiology boosted the credibility of vascular theories. By the time a second edition of his reference book on headache disorders was released posthumously in 1963, migraine was understood as a condition of the vascular system.[57] Wolff's innovative and scientific approach is also generally credited with launching headache as a subspecialty in medicine. In 1959, a small group of physicians founded the American Association for the Study of Headache (AASH, now the American Headache Society); by 1961, they began publishing *Headache*, a scientific journal dedicated to the subject. Similar organizations were founded in the United Kingdom, notably the Migraine Trust, founded in 1965, and in 1981, the International Headache Society (IHS).

Wolff's experiments would have been enough to ensure his place in headache history. But Meyer had taught him that the body responds to emotions and personality. Vascular dilation and constriction might be the mechanism of migraine, but Wolff believed that a close study of personality and emotions would reveal the true cause of migraine. Wolff described the migraine personality as ambitious, successful, perfectionist, and efficient—in other words, a person of good moral character.[58] Wolff believed that these tendencies began in childhood: "The individual with migraine aims to gain approval by doing *more than* and *better than* his fellows through 'application' and 'hard work' and to gain security by holding to a stable environment and a given system of excellent performance, even at high cost of energy. This brings increasing responsibility and admiration, but gains little love, and greater resentment at the pace he feels obliged to maintain. Then the tension associated with repeated frustration, sustained resentment, and growing anxiety is often followed by prostrating fatigue, the setting in which the migraine attack occurs."[59] Wolff, who also had migraine, developed this profile from in-depth psychological interviews with subjects recruited from patients, friends, colleagues, and medical students who experienced migraine.[60] This subject population suffered from a grave selection problem—Wolff recruited subjects from a clinic that attracted professionals who might easily fit into this description. Without a doubt, Wolff also had his own obsessive and perfectionist tendencies in mind.

Wolff's migraine personality was also informed by a burgeoning psychodynamic literature that viewed bodies as "systems of psychobiological adaptations."[61] Using this framework, migraine could be understood to be a protective device that provided a way for the body to withdraw from stressful situations. In fact, migraine was thought to be an especially useful adaptation for overruling an overdetermined, overly ambitious mind. Nevertheless, this psychosomatic framework emphasized the *realness* of migraine. Should any of his students forget that emotions could have as real of an impact as any somatic, measurable fluid, Wolff would remind them. Scrawled on the bottom of his lecture notes were the words "You are at the beginning of a new era when—Loves Hates Fears are as real as management of lump [*sic*] in the chest or pus in the pericardium."[62] Psychosomatic medicine did not, for Wolff, mean "imagined."

Like the nervous temperament before it, the migraine personality had a metaphorical quality that coincided nicely with both the vasomotor theory of migraine and the relatively high socioeconomic status of Wolff's patients. The person with a migraine personality experienced something of a "high" under great stress. When patients failed to meet their own unrealistic expectations, they became tense and fatigued. This model for understanding migraine replicated the migrainous vasculature proposed by Latham: the patient became overly tense, causing vasoconstriction, and then fatigued, causing vasodilation. However, where the nineteenth-century nervous sufferer belonged to the "cultured classes" of England, Wolff's patient was a product and reflection of the newly organized middle class of mid-twentieth-century America. The masculinized patient in Wolff's description could be any "organization man": an executive, a manager, or a mid-level worker. The migraine personality embodied both the capitalist's dreams and anxieties: "Nine-tenths of the migrainous subjects were unusually ambitious and preoccupied with achievement and 'success.' Almost all attempted to dominate their environments—the less successful merely by the force of their demands and the tyranny of their moods, and the more successful through the acquisition of power, money, or distinction."[63]

If, as Foucault argued, modernity was the act of disciplining bodies, then Wolff's migraine personality was discipline in its extreme—a pathological reaction to the corporeal demands of power.[64] His subjects' neatness and fastidiousness, he wrote, was exceeded only by their efficiency. People with migraine loved order and repetition, feared failure, and resented interruptions. They created elaborate "schemes, plans, and ar-

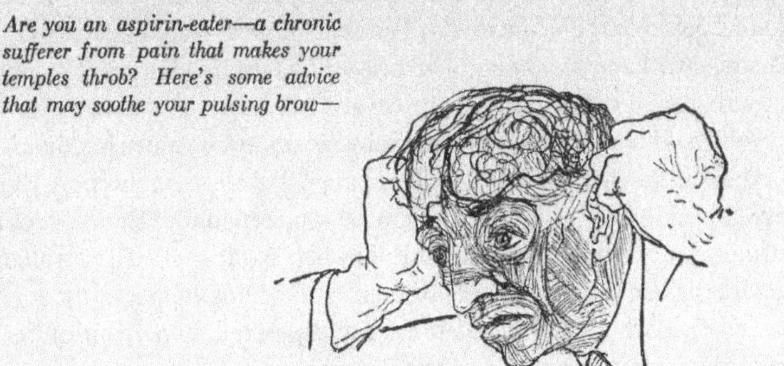

Are you an aspirin-eater—a chronic sufferer from pain that makes your temples throb? Here's some advice that may soothe your pulsing brow—

Headaches Are a Luxury

by HELEN FURNAS

THE KIND of high-pressure big-shot who lives, breathes, eats, drinks, sleeps and dreams his unbridled ambitions has been called a lot of names, few of them complimentary. Now he has a brand new, strictly scientific label—he's a "migraine-type."

all fees are turned back into a research fund—Dr. Wolff has observed hundreds of patients, from captains of industry to humble immigrants, and succeeded in isolating a kind of psychological quirk they have in common that predisposes them to dizzy,

FIGURE 1.2 "Headaches Are a Luxury." Courtesy of Medical Center Archives of NewYork-Presbyterian / Weill Cornell.

rangements," but "had great difficulty in complying with or adapting themselves to systems imposed on them by others." The description of type A personalities varied depending on who had them. Women migraine patients who "worked" at home also wanted everything to be "just so," but they had difficulty delegating even simple household tasks, like dishwashing, to housemaids.[65]

A popular article written about Wolff's migraine personality illustrates this pathologized worker, with a cartoonish man dressed in a business collared shirt, hands on his temple with a stressed, anxious expression. The first paragraph reads "The kind of high-pressure big-shot who lives, breathes, eats, drinks, sleeps and dreams his unbridled ambitions has been called a lot of names, few of them complimentary. Now he has a brand new, strictly scientific label—he's a 'migraine-type'" (see figure 1.2).[66] The headline to that article, "Headaches Are a Luxury," suggested that, at least in the popular imagination, migraine provided a break from work that one could only enjoy if one had enough money. Wolff's advice to these executive workers was similarly luxurious: as a useful migraine preventive measure, take a daily afternoon break and play a game of squash.[67]

Wolff held his male patients in high esteem, even valorizing them. As Goodell put it, "Migraine people [are] almost always sought-after, exemplary citizens—responsible, conscientious and reliable."[68] But the tenor of the migraine personality quickly shifted when Wolff applied it to women.[69] Wolff described the migrainous woman as unwilling to accept the female role, particularly in sexual relations. He described 80 percent of his female sample as sexually dissatisfied. "Orgasm was seldom attained and the sex act was accepted, as at best, a reasonable marital duty. In several instances it was deemed frankly unpleasant and was resented."[70] Furthermore, the migrainous woman was sometimes "reluctant to accept . . . the consequences of maternity."[71] In contrast, Wolff reported that his male patients were sexually well adjusted, even if their sex drive occasionally suffered "as an accompaniment of ambition and hard application to work."[72] Three of Wolff's male patients did experience "sexual maladjustment," but Wolff pointed out that they had "vigorous sex drive[s, but] . . . were married to sexually indifferent or frigid wives."[73] Women, it seems, were always the source of sexual problems.

These passages notwithstanding, Wolff's discussions of women and migraine were intriguingly limited, especially given that by then most physicians had agreed that women experienced migraines more often than men.[74] Much like his Victorian predecessors, Wolff preferred to talk about headache disorders in the masculine. Likewise, his descriptions of migraine emphasized masculine anxieties about the rigors of work life.

However, many other physicians at the time wrote about migraine as a highly feminized women's condition. Articles about women and migraine were dominated by concerns with domestic anxieties and sexual frigidities. This gender bias is most evident in the migraine texts written by Walter C. Alvarez (1884–1978), a gastroenterologist, who, like so many other headache doctors, had migraine, albeit in a quite mild form.[75] Alvarez was a self-proclaimed admirer of Wolff and the first elected treasurer of the newly formed AASH.[76] He worried that so many migrainous women sought diagnostic tests and spent so much money on doctors when doctors had so few effective migraine treatments.[77] The more appropriate role for the physician, he argued, would be to spend time with the patient, "in talking over her life problems and in showing her how to live more calmly and happily, than in making useless examinations."[78] "It is an axiom with me, he added, "that whenever a woman is having three attacks of migraine a week, it means that she is either psychopathic or else she is overworking or worrying or fretting, or otherwise using her brain wrongly."[79] If, for example, the "exciting cause of the attacks is marital infelicity and much thinking about divorce," Alvarez could "almost cure the disease by getting the woman to see clearly that she isn't tough enough or heartless or unkind enough to go ahead and get the divorce she craves. Then when she stops thinking about it she stops having headaches and gets as well as she can be."[80] Of their husbands, he would tell them, "You had to have an angel to put up with all your illnesses and you got him."[81]

Alvarez's depiction of the migrainous woman was reactionary in the degree to which she resembled Victorian descriptions of hysteria and the nervous temperament. These women, "petite, full breasted, and with a nice figure," were full of "intelligence and social charm." He drew attention to "their unusual sensitiveness, their nervous tension, and their easy fatigability." He described them as "tense, quick in thought and movement" and liable to "wilt quickly under any strain." He even evoked the old "wandering womb" paradigm of hysteria, by describing migrainous women as having a "hard myomatous uterus"—which he suggested had something to do with what he alleged were frequent infertility problems found among migrainous women.[82] He argued this, despite the fact that he also agreed that "since 1867, it has been known that the cause of migraine is a hereditary peculiarity of the brain."[83] Alvarez's writing was popular and produced few challenges from other physicians, presumably because his writing captured one school of thought in the headache community at the time. (See figure 1.3 for a depiction of a female migraine patient in a 1960s pharmaceutical advertisement.)

By the 1960s, the scope of psychiatry in headache medicine had ballooned. A widely read classification system of headache disorders, published in 1962, characterized almost all primary headaches as psychosomatic: "Essential in the study of headache, in most instances, is an appraisal of its close link to the patient's situation, activities, and attitudes. Sometimes in obvious ways, more often in subtle ones, headache may be the *principal manifestation of temporary or sustained difficulties in life adjustment.*"[84] This approach maintained that any vascular changes were secondary to psychological conditions.

By the late 1960s, it seemed as though psychology was the only lens through which to understand migraine. Consider, for example, a session

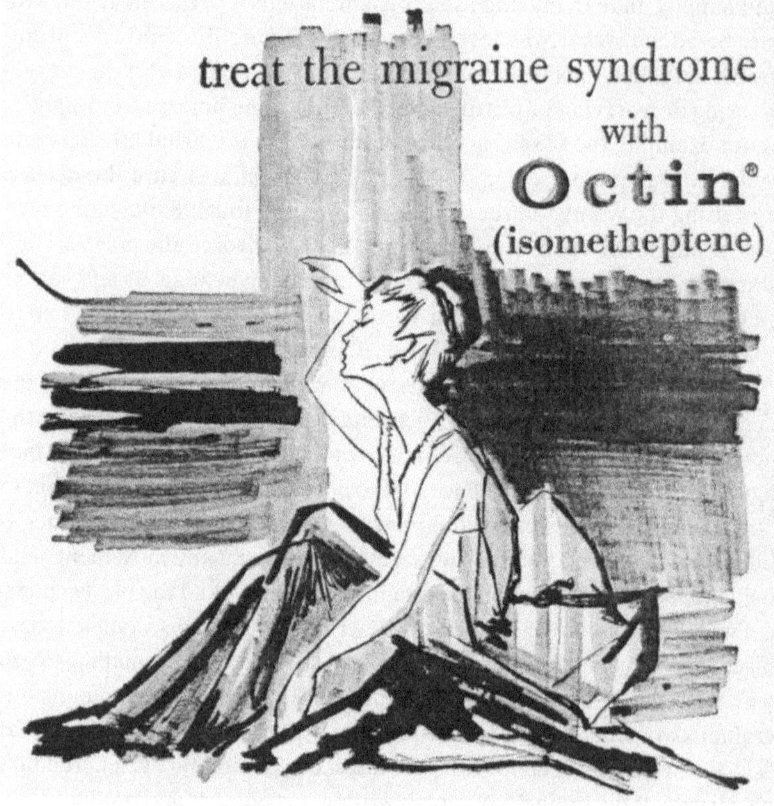

FIGURE 1.3 1960s Pharmaceutical advertisement from 1960s journal *Headache.*

on the "Psychiatric Aspects of Headache" at the 1967 meeting of the AASH.[85] The first speaker on the panel, Harry Garner, chairman of the Department of Neurology and Psychiatry at the Chicago Medical School, argued that "the crucial factor for migraine . . . is intense rage."[86] Indeed, he argued that those with "intense, unbearable, continuous headache who are unresponsive to the usual analgesic medications for days at a time" (read: those he could not treat) had "violent rage reactions of a *homicidal* nature."[87] As for those with lesser headache, he suggested that they "permit hostility and irritability displays within the limits permitted by the excuse 'I have a headache.'"[88] The second speaker, Bernard Shulman, assistant professor of psychiatry at Northwestern University and chairman of the Department of Psychiatry of St. Joseph's Hospital in Chicago, essentially agreed with Dr. Garner. And the third speaker, Perry S. MacNeal, soon-to-be president of the AASH and associate professor of clinical medicine at the University of Pennsylvania Medical School, made two additional suggestions.

> There is a standard question that I ask of all patients whom I suspect of having migraine, and that is "How many times have you gone to bed at night and left the dirty dishes in the sink?" If the lady can say to this honestly, "Oh, I do it once in awhile," she simply does not have migraine, she has some other kind of headache. If she says, "Oh, I never do that doctor" then I follow it up and say, "Do you mean to tell me that when you have one of these blinding headaches, you can't see and you're vomiting, you will do those dishes?" and she will say "Yes, doctor, of course." So it is part of our treatment to always prescribe a sink with two drains so she can vomit in one side and do dishes in the other.[89]

MacNeal's sense of humor belies his insistence on adhering to a highly gendered personality-oriented theory of migraine. MacNeal would rather reconsider his diagnosis of migraine than question whether the so-called migraine personality might occasionally fail to describe his patient population. Garner, Shulman, and MacNeal painted a very bleak mental portrait of the migraine patient, indeed.

How did psychological theories come this far in migraine medicine? Judy Segal has argued that the explanatory power and popularity of the migraine personality could be attributed to its expansiveness—the migraine personality could describe almost anyone.[90] The migraine personality became what Ian Hacking refers to as an "interactive kind."[91] Interactive kinds are categories that not only define but also constitute people. That is, some classifications organize individuals' experiences in such a way that they adapt or respond to their classification. Such was the case with the migraine personality. People with migraine began to adapt to Wolff's concept of the "migraine personality": the category altered how they thought, behaved, and classified themselves. That the category was expansive allowed even the most frazzled and disorganized of migraine patients to argue that they, too, had a migraine personality.

Joan Didion, for example, found the migraine personality compelling despite its failure to describe her at all. When a doctor told her that she didn't look like a migraine personality because her hair was messy, he followed, "But I suppose you're a compulsive housekeeper." She demurred:

"Actually my house is kept even more negligently than my hair, but the doctor was right nonetheless: perfectionism can also take the form of spending most of a week writing and rewriting and not writing a single paragraph."[92] Didion did the hard work for the doctor. She located the one area of her personality in which she thought she might have compulsive, obsessive, or perfectionist tendencies. By adjusting her sense of self to fit her doctor's notion of the migraine personality, she behaved just as Hacking described how an interactive kind might.

The Fall of the Vasomotor-Psychosomatic Paradigm

Wolff's vasomotor-psychosomatic paradigm dominated migraine medicine from the 1930s to the early 1970s. But its failure was heralded in 1962, when pharmaceutical giant Sandoz (now Novartis) received Food and Drug Administration (FDA) approval to sell methysergide, a drug that could reduce the number of migraine attacks in some patients. Methysergide, a derivative of ergotamine, was too dangerous to be widely used. Like its forebearer, the psychedelic lysergic acid diethylamide-25 (LSD)—a drug also created in Sandoz's laboratories—methysergide could cause hallucinations, insomnia, and disorders of high cerebral function, as well as vasomotor and fibrotic problems. But its efficacy as a *preventative* drug suggested a new theory of migraine. Methysergide worked by altering serotonin levels instead of by regulating the vascular system. In response to the drug's effectiveness, researchers began to reframe migraine as a serotonergic, and therefore biochemical, problem.[93]

The embrace of biochemical approaches meant the corresponding rejection of psychogenic theories. Reflecting on this effect, Neil Raskin wrote: "I was still in training when methysergide was introduced in 1960. It was quite astonishing how this drug changed physicians' thinking about the nature of migraine. Prior to that time . . . migraine was thought to be predominantly psychosomatic. . . . Suddenly, patients could take a few tablets of methysergide and within a week they were headache free. No change in their internal milieu. Cured."[94] That the efficacy of a medication should erode a psychosomatic theory is not surprising. This is a fairly common phenomenon. Several disorders understood to be psychosomatic (depression or stomach ulcers, for example) were reframed as somatic with the discovery of effective medication.[95] Yet in the case of migraine, ergotamine derivatives had been used successfully to treat the disorder for thirty-five years, yet had given a boost to theories of migraine as psychosomatic. Why did ergotamine promote psychosomatic theories, while methysergide eroded them? The answer is that methysergide worked as a preventative, eliminating migraines without changing the temperament of the patient. Raskin suggests this was an unexpected outcome when he says, "within a week they were headache free. No change in their internal milieu."

With the discovery that serotonin might play a central role in the pathophysiology of migraine, a few headache researchers began to question the existence and clinical usefulness of the migraine personality. Australian neurologist James Lance published the first serious critique in the 1960s when he wrote that Wolff's observations were mere clinical impressions and ought not be generalized to the population: "In the absence of published control groups of similar age, sex, social and economic background, it would be unwise to attach too much importance to [the migraine personality]. In asking students attending lectures whether they would consider themselves as showing similar obsessional trends or anxiety symptoms [as are found in the migraine personality], the author has been impressed that about half the group think they do. Possibly their less obsessional brethren do not turn up for lectures. Alternatively, migrainous patients may simply mirror the world around them."[96] W. E. Waters followed with one of the first population-based epidemiological studies of migraine.[97] He concluded that the migraine personality finding was merely a quirk of selection bias. People with migraine from the professional classes simply sought help from their physicians more often than their working-class counterparts. Others, like Alick Elithorn, noted that descriptions of the migraine personality had become so broad as to include almost every personality characteristic: "In practice, the variety of temperament traits which it is claimed are correlated with the liability to migraine are almost as numerous as the physicians who take a primarily psychodynamic approach."[98]

Nevertheless, the migraine personality remained a regular feature of medical writing through the 1970s and 1980s, despite convincing evidence that debunked the idea. For example, in 1973, Seymour Diamond and Donald Dalessio, then codirectors of the famous Diamond Headache Clinic in Chicago, wrote that the inability of people with migraine to adapt represents the repressed hostility of the migraine patient.[99] In their 1978 book for patients, *Freedom from Headaches*, Joel Saper, medical director of the prestigious Michigan Head-Pain and Neurological Institute, and his coauthor Kenneth Magee wrote that the "so-called migraine personality is characterized by compulsive, perfectionistic, and self-critical tendencies. Often these features reflect an upbringing that placed a high premium on discipline, restraint, achievement, and respect for authority."[100] Although they say that the migraine personality is a "matter of debate," their book includes a "migraine personality quiz . . . for [the readers'] entertainment."[101]

Even when reviewing a literature that seemingly could not support the migraine personality, researchers continued to write about the importance of assessing emotional and personality factors in migraine. Russell Packard, a psychologist who had written a great deal about migraine, made exactly this sort of counterintuitive suggestion in a 1979 article published in *Headache.* Even after discussing Arnold Friedman's 1958 observation that "no one personality type could describe all migraine patients," Packard argued that "these emotional and personality factors in migraine are important to determine when taking a patient's history because they may be helpful in treatment. For example, a migraineur who gets headaches only on weekends because he 'loses his structure of the week,' often can be helped by simply having him plan some weekend activities in advance, so he doesn't wake up Saturday morning with a headache to fill his 'unplanned' day."[102]

The supposedly defunct migraine personality persists even in the new millennium. For example, even contemporary reference books that purport to refute psychosomatic medicine contain modified versions of the migraine personality. The 2001 edition of *Wolff's Headache and Other Head Pain* states: "Behavioral issues are not a popular topic to discuss with headache patients. For years, the belief that headache disorders were caused by an unstable constitution or psychiatric illness stigmatized people with headache. Although we have come a long way since then . . . behavioral issues must be examined. . . . Behaviors with potential for negative impact on health include Type A behaviors, a generalized high-intensity approach to life, self-sacrificing behaviors, negative cognitive styles, overly high self-expectations, behaviors that contribute to difficulties in work or personal relationships, passivity, and lack of initiative."[103] Here, the tension is between the "stigmatizing" "belief" that headache disorders are "caused" by an "unstable constitution" and the authors' insistence that behaviors *must* be examined as a potential contributor to headache disorders. The authors ask colleagues to examine patients for the same psychological problems that defined the original migraine personality despite a lack of evidence that such problems exist. Their list of behaviors to watch for remains as expansive as the original migraine personality: type A behaviors, a high-intensity approach to life, and overly high self-expectations are somehow linked to passivity and lack of initiative. Almost anyone could fall into this range of behavioral pathology.

Psychological explanations of migraine remain an extraordinarily popular trope in self-help books for migraine care. Take, for example, the most popular self-help book on this topic, *Heal Your Headache: The 1.2.3 Program*, by David Buchholz, a neurologist from Johns Hopkins School of Medicine. Buchholz recommends a strict treatment protocol for migraine prevention, which includes the immediate removal of all abortive drugs (i.e., the drugs that one takes to interrupt a migraine); a strict diet; and, if all else fails, preventive medications. The treatment plan is difficult to follow—he suggests that people quit taking their pain medications "cold turkey" without help from a physician, lest "you and your doctor . . . become entangled in a sticky web of victimization, dependence, blame and guilt . . . quick fixes . . . [that] undermine your determination to do what you can to prevent migraine."[104] If his methods do not work, Buchholz observes, "sometimes it's hard to let go."[105] He confides that he is pessimistic about patients who are "entrenched in or seeking disability status, or pursuing a lawsuit, based on headaches."[106] Illness behavior, he explains, can help motivate migraine, as "when we're sick, others give us their attention, concern, affection, sympathy, help, forgiveness, and permission to be excused from work and other responsibilities . . . our subconscious may have some other hidden agenda that interferes with response to treatment."[107]

Buchholz relies most heavily on psychological explanations of migraine when his recommendations fail to work for the patient. For him, the next obvious explanation is that the fault lies in the psyche of the person who *refuses* to get better. But it's also important to remember that Buchholz isn't talking about just *any* kind of person. He's implicitly describing a feminized patient, one who could easily become involved in "victimization, dependence, blame and guilt." Buchholz's use of the psyche as a last-ditch explanatory model for the difficult patient underscores one remaining way that biomedicine manages the balance between mind and body in migraine: when patients—especially female patients—become "difficult," the psyche remains a convenient explanation for treatment failure.

Entering a Neurobiological Age

Buchholz's perspective is now the exception rather than the rule. All across medicine, disorders once thought to be psychological are now considered to be diseases of a "broken brain."[108] Biological psychiatry has replaced psychodynamic models in American psychiatry.[109] Explanatory models that once emphasized abstract psychic phenomena, like personality and early-life conflict, have given way to a singular focus on neural pathways. A dysfunctional brain is now seen as the source of conditions as varied as depression, schizophrenia, social anxiety disorder, autism, and obsessive-compulsive behavior. Pharmaceuticals have, by and large, replaced talk therapy. This "new style of thought," explains sociologist Nikolas Rose, has completely altered how we think of mind and body, so that "mind is simply what the brain does."[110]

As medicine goes, so goes migraine.

The notion that migraine could be a purely vascular disorder is now considered by most headache specialists to be "untenable."[111] Instead, they now argue that migraine should be considered a *neurovascular* phenomenon. In this model, the activation of the trigeminal nervous system results in the dilation of blood vessels, which, in turn, results in pain and further nerve activation.[112] Contemporary neurologists have revived the nerve-storm theory of Edward Liveing, whom they often claim as their rightful predecessor.[113] Efforts to understand the pathophysiology of migraine at a molecular level are oriented toward locating potential "targets" for pharmacological intervention. Migraine is now a major economic market worth billions of dollars.

Following American psychiatry's lead, headache specialists have reduced mental aspects of migraine to the body. Wolff's theories about "personality" have given way to epidemiological studies of psychological comorbidity, particularly with depression and anxiety. The concept of comorbidity allows researchers to argue that some forms of mental illness have a greater than random possibility of occurring in an individual with migraine, without suggesting a reason why this might be the case. This research has demonstrated that a person with migraine is more likely than a person without migraine to have depression or anxiety (and vice versa), while remaining agnostic on the causal direction. The two disorders could share a biological cause, like a genetic predisposition or an environmental trigger. Or as many headache advocates point out, living with migraine could cause depression or anxiety. While far fewer stakeholders maintain that the opposite could be true, depression is thought to worsen (although not cause) migraine.

The language of comorbidity is meant to be more biologically "correct," but it serves other purposes as well. For physicians, comorbidity serves to isolate the disease that is most of interest to them, while marginalizing other disorders. For patients, comorbidity allows migraine to be distinguished as a disease quite distinct from psychological problems—a maneuver that may feel like it protects the person with migraine from defamation of moral character. And yet, the basic description of the migraine population has remained the same. Not only are people with migraine thought to be more likely than people without migraine to have depression or anxiety, mental illness is thought to be endemic within clinical migraine populations. As a result, headache specialists continue to hire psychiatrists, psychologists, and other behavioral health workers; new patients are screened using the Minnesota Multiphasic Personality Inventory; and migraine continues to be treated, with some efficacy, with drugs typically used for and associated with depression.[114] At the same time, headache doctors find that they must persistently reassure their patients that these psychoactive drugs and psychological tests have nothing to do with their mental state or moral character. As one might imagine, this is tricky. Making this balancing act even trickier is the problematic fact that many of the conditions with which migraine is comorbid, like depression and anxiety, are themselves highly gendered, deeply feminized, and come burdened with their own set of cultural baggage.

Moral Character in the Neurobiological Age

After Susan Sontag had her first bout with cancer, she wrote a famous essay called "Illness as Metaphor" that forcefully rejected the various cultural mythologies that surround diseases.[115] Illness, she argued, was too often cloaked in mystifying metaphors. Cancer was not, as it was often described in the 1970s, a "punishment" that happened to people with controlling personalities; tuberculosis had nothing to do with artistic soulfulness or nobility, as nineteenth-century novels presented it; and AIDS ought not be considered a "plague" that "punishes" those who engage in morally inappropriate behavior. To use such metaphors served only to heap additional and unnecessary suffering on the patient. Her suggested cure was to purify all diseases of any metaphorical thinking whatsoever; to remain true to a scientific discourse that regards disease as, simply, a disease.

By reducing the mind to empirically measurable parts of the body, headache specialists are, in effect, trying to do just as Sontag recommended. Her vision resonates with a commonsense understanding of how science and culture operate. According to this logic, objective science ought to eradicate cultural biases, like the sexist assumptions that were embedded in the psychosomatic theories of migraine that were so popular in the twentieth century. But as many have pointed out, this commonsense understanding does not stand up to scrutiny. For one thing, as George Lakoff and Mark Johnson demonstrated, we think through metaphor.[116] Metaphor is, by necessity, always shaping our language and thought. Investigating migraine through a historical lens, as I have done here, reminds us that medicine, metaphor, and meaning are intrinsically linked. The issue is not whether to use metaphors, but which metaphors to use. In the next chapter, I explore both how metaphor has shaped contemporary headache medicine and, in particular, the extent to which contemporary headache doctors have been able to free themselves from the yoke of psychosomatic medicine and all of its attendant meanings.

CHAPTER TWO

All in Her Brain

My research on headache disorders began in 2001 with a trip to the International Headache Congress in New York City. Given my previous experiences as a migraine patient, I half-expected to hear headache specialists laughing at neurotic patients who monopolized their time with inane complaints about pain. What I didn't expect to see was the New York Hilton decked out with large brains. There were brains everywhere. Scientific discussions were punctuated with PET scans and MRIs of the brain during a migraine. Images of brains illustrated the scientific literature displayed in the exhibit hall. Large brains were projected onto conference space walls. Brains loomed on the large banners that advertised organizations. Free-floating brains dominated, but brains were visible even in portrayals of patients, many of whom had transparent heads. The brain-shaped swag distributed to doctors by headache organizations and pharmaceutical companies included candy "gummy brains," squeezable brains for stress, brain-shaped lapel pins, and a "virtual brain map" on CD-ROM.

I found the images encouraging—it all seemed so scientific. Prior to this, I had only seen headache disorders represented with images of patients—typically women—some with hands pressed to their foreheads, supposedly in pain; others beaming happily because they had just taken a pill that made them feel better. So it surprised me that the brain was being used as synecdoche for migraine. Beyond the visual motif, it seemed like everyone at the conference was having the same conversation, and that conversation focused on brains. In headache medicine, migraine had undergone a paradigmatic transformation from a disorder of the mind to a disorder of the brain.

As my research proceeded, the brain, and its implications for migraine's legitimacy, became a constant theme in my conversations with headache specialists. Take this exchange, for example. During a conference break, I sat down for a cup of coffee with a headache specialist who had held many leadership positions in headache organizations. Gesturing toward the brains that hung on the walls around us, I asked, "What has it meant for migraine that it has undergone this transformation from a condition of the mind to one of the brain?" His reply was a version of one I would hear many times over the years: "The emergence of neuroscience has made migraine a more legitimate condition to treat. It means that it is real."

The brain is much more than just the object of study for headache specialists; it is also a talisman that they have invested with the power to bring a new legitimacy to their field. Like all talismans, it comes with a myth. For headache specialists, the brain and the neurobiological turn it symbolizes represent a key moment in the evolution of their field. For example, addressing a large audience at the 2002 annual conference of the American Headache Society (AHS), the premier organization for headache professionals in the United States, neurologist David Dodick made a common distinction between past and present practices in headache medicine: "Previously, we told all our patients that it's all in your head and you should relax. In fact, it *is* all in their head; it's in their brain" (fieldnotes). Headache can now be taken seriously, specialists tell each other and the world, because it's no longer a condition of the mind, but a disorder of the brain.

The cultural contestations surrounding migraine profoundly shape headache medicine as a profession and as a body of knowledge. Headache specialists often blame the prominence of psychosomatic medicine in the "bad old days" to account for what they see as the problems of "legitimacy" that continue to dog their field. Headache medicine, they claim—like the disorder it treats—has never been taken seriously despite being a serious business. Its long-running failure to provide effective treatments and its popular association with difficult, psychologically brittle patients has made it a low-status field. But their concerns extend beyond psychosomatism and toward gender. They worried that women with migraine appeared in both medical texts and cultural representations as weak, oversensitive, and neurotic. In this context, headache specialists' focus on neuroreduction—a reframing of migraine that reduces migraine to the biology of the brain—is hardly genderless. The brain presents a fantasy in which headache specialists can somehow circumvent the embodied and often difficult patients in their clinics.

This chapter analyzes this narrative of progress with the ultimate goal of assessing headache specialists' claim that neuroscience has revolutionized migraine. In the end, I argue that the neuroreduction of headache medicine has thus far failed to be the transformative development that the headache community believes it to be and which it so craves. Headache medicine's problems with legitimacy persist despite the "discovery" of a neurobiological mechanism underlying migraine. For while the emphasis on the brain does somewhat mitigate migraine's association with psychosomatic, feminized personalities, locating migraine in the brain also managed to inscribe gendered cultural assumptions about the personalities of headache patients into the physical structure of their bodies. The newly biomedicalized migraine has not eliminated characterizations of a migraine patient as a particular kind of person, but instead has transformed the moral character of the migraine patient into a new, still highly gendered biomedical configuration.

The Legitimacy Deficit

In order to understand the neurobiological turn in migraine, one must first understand that headache specialists have always had trouble convincing others that their work is worthwhile and meaningful.[1] The epigraph to Edward Liveing's 1873 landmark treatise on megrim, for example, quotes an even older treatise, written in 1849, by the eminent physiologist Marshall Hall: "Nothing is so common—nothing is viewed as of such trifling import—as the seizure termed 'Sick headache.' Yet I have known Sick-headache issue in paroxysmal attacks of a very severe nature, both apopleptic and epileptic."[2] In 1953 the British physician Nevil Leyton was still complaining that migraine "has received scant attention from the medical profession down the ages. . . . Perhaps the explanation lies in the fact that it is still considered by so many to be 'just a headache.'"[3] Again and again, headache specialists have lamented what they see as the yawning gap between the intense suffering caused by head pain and the attitudes of the medical profession or culture more broadly, who consider it to be trivial, "trifling," and unworthy of serious attention or concern.

At the beginning of the twenty-first century, headache specialists still report a legitimacy deficit. Migraine, headache specialists believe, is taken far less seriously than it ought to be given the burden it places on patients and society writ large. Headache specialists' struggles in closing this deficit emerged as a constant theme in conference proceedings, corridor talk, interviews, and even in published medical literature. So important is the issue of legitimacy to headache specialists that the AHS named "legitimacy" the theme of its fiftieth anniversary. Alongside a conference devoted to this theme, the organization distributed a corresponding issue of *Headache*, its official journal, on the subject of "Legitimacy." The editor, John Rothrock, kicked off the issue with an editorial that recalled that "within my demi generation of neurologists, migraine was largely an afterthought, a condition implicitly (or explicitly) 'psychosomatic' at which we might throw a bit of therapeutic this n' that: a beta blocker here, an oral ergotamine there and—for the more adventuresome—the occasional infusion of dihydroergotamine."[4]

Discussions about the legitimacy deficit were not limited to anniversaries—leaders spoke about legitimacy problems at every opportunity. For example, when accepting an award, Seymour Solomon, a senior headache specialist, laughed about a time early in his career when famed neurologist Arnold Friedman asked him to join his premier headache unit at Montefiore Medical Center, which was then "the only game in town and . . . indeed the only game in the country." Even though patients had to wait six months to see a doctor, Solomon says he turned Friedman down because "I was interested in organic disease and not in neurotic symptoms of women, which was the concept of headache at that time." He did, eventually, agree to join Friedman's clinic once the etiological framing of "headache evolved from psychogenic to biogenic" (fieldnotes).

Solomon's comments point to an ongoing concern among headache specialists: the need to distance their specialty from psychosomatic medicine, in general, and a perception that they treat only neurotic women, in particular. Many agreed with the specialist who told me in an interview, "there's been too much mind associated with the issue of headache, putting [it] into more of a psychological bailiwick than it belonged." Another specialist blamed mentors, arguing that if "most neurologists" think their patients are, "you know, psychosomatic, depressed, anxious," then "that stigma, of course, when that's all you hear from your mentors and your teachers, um, you know that has an impact and so a lot of the residents would feel the same way. They sort of imprinted a stigma on these patients and went in with sort of a, I don't want to say a bad attitude, but went in with an attitude that needed to be readjusted. So they went in jaded and came out jaded" (interview). The problem was widely framed as a lingering aftertaste of psychosomatic medicine

These general comments, however, suggest some conceptual slippage between the categories of "psychosomatic patients" and "women." Headache specialists often told me, for example, that their colleagues had a low opinion of migraine and migraine patients; often they shrugged off migraine patients, saying, "Oh yeah, this is just a headache. This is just someone who can't cope" (fieldnotes). Doctors, they said, perceive headache patients as difficult or unpleasant and "just whiny" (fieldnotes). But "difficult" patients weren't just any patients. As one put it, "I think that women get discriminated against. I, I still hear that from some of my colleagues about how their women patients whine, you know all this stuff." Another headache specialist told me: "The association with [migraine] has been that this is a psychological disorder of women and it's been a way in which traditional jokes about not tonight, dear, . . . with headache, um, as disorder associated with women as an excuse not to have sex with their husband or not to visit their in-laws or not to attend various functions, things of that sort. I think that's been a very negative image that has been associated with women and migraine." In short, headache specialists worry that nonspecialists perceive headache patients as having highly gendered personality problems. They are difficult, hypochondriacal, and resistant to treatment. These observations find support among surveys of nonspecialists. In one study of general neurologists, a quarter of those surveyed agreed with the following statement: "Many headache patients have motivation to maintain their disability."[5]

To headache specialists, it seems that these concerns about the legitimacy of headache patients create problems for their professional status through long-established practices of training, employment, and renumeration. One neurologist, for instance, told me in an interview, "Headache is still not a popular specialty. You can take a thousand neurologists and you will maybe get 10 percent of them to admit that they don't mind seeing a patient with headache." This specialist's 10 percent figure may not be hyperbole. Membership in professional societies—if this may serve as a proxy for physicians' disease-specific interests—reveals even less interest in headache medicine than that. Only a thousand neurologists count themselves as members of the AHS in comparison to twenty thousand neurologists who are members of the American Academy of Neurology

(AAN).[6] Fifty years after the AHS was founded, headache specialists continue to lament the "lofty disdain many clinicians hold for that condition [migraine]."[7]

Headache disorders are not a required part of most medical school curriculums, despite the fact that headache is one of the most common symptoms presented to doctors. Formal training, when offered in medical schools, is quite limited—surveys estimate that US undergraduate medical programs spend anywhere between two to four hours of undergraduate training on headache disorders.[8] A 2005 study by Maya Kommineni and Alan Finkel revealed that only 31 percent of neurology department chairs and residency training directors believe that headache is adequately taught in medical school.[9]

Of course, very little of residents' education is formal; most of it occurs informally in the ward. Nonetheless, the neurologists who convened at AHS conferences thought the lack of formal education perpetuated headache's status problems among their colleagues. Several headache specialists complained about this systematic disinterest in headache disorders. As one headache specialist put it: "I think that when you have a disorder as common as migraine and related disorders and you have, and at least in the past, such limited exposure to it in medical school training and residency training, that essentially unless you take the time to study it on your own, you come out with a sense that it may not be an important disorder and worthy of recognition and treatment. . . . I think that residents get exposure to the rarest of disorders that may cause headache and not to the most common" (interview). Similarly, Peter Goadsby, a prominent headache specialist, noted that "headache is the commonest symptom found in neurologic outpatients—and, paradoxically, the least taught to neurology residents. It's like training electricians, but not telling them about light bulbs."[10]

Headache specialists argue that because their work is devalued within neurology, jobs are often difficult to come by. They claim that many neurology departments do not feel it necessary to hire a dedicated headache specialist. I met dozens of physicians who said that although they had "no special training" in headache treatment, they had been named the de facto headache specialist in their clinic because they were the only ones who "didn't mind seeing headache patients" (fieldnotes).[11] Surveys of physicians' attitudes toward migraine support the anecdotal evidence that neurology departments do indeed marginalize headache patients. Despite the fact that most department chairs believe that migraine is, in fact, a "legitimate" brain disorder, general neurologists complain that treating migraine patients is time-consuming and that these patients tend to have psychological problems.[12]

I found it difficult to make sense of this lack of jobs. On the one hand, the widespread contempt felt by physicians for headache patients has created a niche market for the specialist willing to take them on. One headache specialist joked to me during an interview that most of her colleagues "just want to kiss my feet that I'm willing to see the headache patients. . . . It's like, you know, they're glad, you know, 'Don't leave! We don't want to see those patients!' " (interview). Indeed, it was partly the marginalization of headache patients that motivated the creation of clinics that specialized in headache treatment. As a 1971 article in the journal *Headache* explained: "Though most practicing physicians are called upon to treat headaches, few are enthralled by their experience. In fact, most physicians would rather refer to a colleague a patient with persistent intractable headache. In the United States, Headache Clinics are rare, but those that do exist attract a large clientele soon after their establishment and relieve many hard-pressed physicians of some of their burdensome and time-consuming patients."[13] Headache specialists remain in high demand. For example, as of 2012, the United Council for Neurologic Subspecialties had only board-certified 416 headache specialists, which is a very low number considering that 1–3 percent of American adults are estimated to have chronic migraine.[14]

On the other hand, providing services to headache patients—no matter how needed they are—is often described as a money-losing proposition. The problem is twofold: headache medicine requires few procedures, while at the same time, necessitates long doctor-patient appointments. This matters because in the United States reimbursement rates pay much higher dividends for procedures than "evaluation and management." While other neurological specialties regularly use procedures like electroencephalography (EEG), angiograms, biopsies, and brain imaging techniques, most diagnostics in headache medicine draw on a detailed and lengthy patient history. This is part of why headache patients are regarded as unusually demanding of resources and time. But the problems are multiplied because much headache care happens by telephone in between appointments, since drugs need constant tweaking. Staffing costs, especially paying nurses to answer phones and negotiate with insurance, cut into earning potential. The Food and Drug Administration's 2010 approval of Botox, a drug administered via an expensive procedure, is improving these financial calculations, but in general, financial constraints may make neurology departments hesitant to set aside special resources for headache medicine.[15]

Headache specialists thus find themselves very much sought after, but not well respected or highly paid. Other pain doctors have found themselves in a similar position. Sociologist Isabelle Baszanger has described how pain doctors in France built a specialty out of treating patients cast off by other physicians. Her respondents reported that theirs were "the patients that they [other doctors] no longer know what to do with," or were "no longer desirable." Pain doctors defined their role in the hospital as "rendering a service" by treating the patients whom nobody else could help. But treating stigmatized patients comes at a cost, since pain doctors reported having to work hard to avoid "being taken for cranks."[16] Sociologist Kristin Barker has described how some rheumatologists—another marginalized specialty in medicine—seek to distance themselves from patients with fibromyalgia, even though these patients flood their waiting rooms.[17]

The fact is that treating marginalized patients confers very little occupational prestige. Baszanger notes that there seemed to be a "homology of status" between pain patients and pain doctors.[18] The headache specialists that I observed noted the same phenomenon. As one headache specialist warned me, "headache neurologists are kind of the dowdy wearing lowest caste of neurologists. To stand up and say that you are interested in headache is a chance for you to be stigmatized as a neurologist. You should be aware of that" (interview). One joke I heard while hanging around headache specialists encapsulated their general dissatisfaction: "Headache is the Rodney Dangerfield of medical maladies—it gets no respect."[19]

Studies of prestige hierarchies in medicine have found that medical specialties that deal with diseases associated with the mind are afforded lower prestige. Such studies consistently find that surgical fields, like neurosurgery, are ranked highest, followed closely by internal medicine specialties like cardiology and neurology, while psychiatry is nearly always at the bottom.[20] Most of these studies have focused their attention on prestige hierarchies among specialties, but one study found that doctors could also rank diseases on a prestige hierarchy. Researchers Dag Album and Steinar Westin, for instance, offered physicians and medical students a list of thirty-eight diseases selected to represent a cross section of patients, affected organs, curability rates, and whether the disease was chronic or acute.[21] Doctors ranked highest diseases located in the upper parts of the body or in organs with significant social value in human life. This was particularly the case for such lethal afflictions as myocardial infarction and brain tumor. Diseases without objective markers and which were thought of as problems of the mind were low in prestige (for example, fibromyalgia ranked last in this list), as were those associated with questionable moral character, such as hepatic cirrhosis and AIDS. Three of the lowest ranking diseases (depressive neurosis, anxiety neurosis, and fibromyalgia) were also diseases that disproportionately affect women. Although migraine was not included in the list, the chronic nature of the disorder, its lack of fatality, its association with the mind, and its prevalence among women all suggest that it would likely receive a low ranking.[22]

Over time, I realized that headache specialists were describing to me the multiple ways in which the status and legitimacy of their field were entangled with what they study. First off, pain—the very subject of headache specialists' expertise—is often ignored, marginalized, and misunderstood. What use is there in being an authority on a disorder considered trivial—one that doesn't even kill people!—or, worse, not even "real?" Second, clinical uncertainty is high when treating chronic headache patients. The failure of those with chronic ailments to recover deflates physicians' efforts who, after all, have typically gone into medicine to heal their patients. This in itself might not be problematic, since many high-prestige diseases, like fatal brain tumors, lack effective treatments. But the constant refrain of seeing the same patients return to the clinic, dissatisfied with their treatments, is made more complicated by this last issue: headache specialists argued that their patients were widely understood to be undesirable, stereotypically difficult women—whiny, depressed, and neurotic. They claimed that mere association with their patients diminished their professional status. In short, headache specialists seemed to be suffering from what Erving Goffman referred to as a "courtesy stigma."[23] If patients are stigmatized by a broad public perception that migraine is a condition of psychologically compromised, weak women, then so were their doctors. The trick, then, would be to eliminate this morally compromised person from the clinical encounter. But how could headache specialists treat migraine without treating so-called difficult patients?

The Neurobiological Turn

If headache specialists recognize that their work is not taken seriously because the disorders they treat are themselves not taken seriously, the flip side of this is that headache medicine's search for recognition as a legitimate subspecialty has taken place, as the headache specialist Alan Finkel notes, "simultaneous with the drive to ensure the acceptance of headache disorders as 'real diseases.'"[24] In other words, headache specialists acknowledge that their credibility depends on the credibility of the objects of their expertise. They understand that experts don't just judge the quality of wine or gold or whatever widget is under their purview; they themselves are judged by the status of that which falls within their jurisdiction.[25]

For doctors, as historian Charles Rosenberg has shown, establishing the legitimacy of a disease has historically involved proving it to be a "specific disease," that is, "a biopathological phenomenon with a characteristic mechanism and a predictable course," which is understood to exist independently of its embodiment in any particular patient.[26] Research funding, successful insurance claims, hospital cost management, bureaucratic institutional negotiations, and broader social approval all depend on tracing a set of symptoms to a specific, underlying somatic mechanism whose causal role can be demonstrated using such seemingly objective instruments as laboratory findings and imaging technologies. As a result, many researchers investigating disorders that occupy the border territories between mind and body have limited their scope of inquiry to the body to improve the reliability and legitimacy of their results. This is particularly true in psychiatry, a field in which, as sociologist Nikolas Rose has shown, psychoanalysis has been supplanted by neurobiological explanations focusing on organic dysfunctions of the brain.

Like psychiatrists, headache specialists have attempted to legitimate their subject by transforming it into a biological disorder of the brain. Indeed, the effects of non-neurobiological factors are increasingly discussed only in terms of their impact on the brain. Stress, diet, sex hormones, changes in barometric pressure, bright lights, strong smells, changes in sleeping patterns, alcohol, physical exertion, dehydration, and low blood sugar have all been relegated to the status of migraine "triggers" that activate neuronal processes in the brain. Broader cultural or environmental factors—such as poverty or unemployment—or psychological factors are only of interest in as much as they can be reconfigured into neurobiological accounts of headache disorders. "Reality," as constituted by medical neurobiology, is thus an example of what Emily Martin has called "neuroreductionism," in which the harder-to-quantify effects of individual bodies, society, history, mind, and culture are stripped out to establish the universality and certainty that brings legitimacy.[27] Neuroreductionist thinking promotes a dualism in which the brain is primary and everything else is secondary.

The history of the neurobiological turn in headache medicine demonstrates how closely linked this epistemological shift is to a larger politics of legitimacy. One can trace this history by following the changing dynamics of the AHS over the decades. Founded in 1959, the American Association for the Study of Headache (AAHS), as the AHS was then known, brought together the expertise of doctors from a range of different specialties, including internal medicine, psychiatry, allergy, obstetrics and gynecology, otolaryngology, as well as neurology. The late 1970s and early 1980s, however, were marked by a number of jurisdictional contests between neurologists who began to challenge the vascular and psychosomatic basis of headache medicine—a paradigm that was upheld by the internal medicine physicians who dominated the leadership of the AASH at that time.[28]

Neurologists eventually triumphed and took over the leadership of headache medicine, but, ironically, this was not originally territory that they desired. Drs. John Graham and Seymour Diamond, who were both internal medicine physicians on AASH's board, *invited* neurologists into the leadership. Throughout the 1970s, Graham and Diamond had repeatedly approached neurologist Arnold Friedman about joining the organization. Friedman's resistance posed a credibility problem for AASH; not only was Friedman the director of a pioneering headache unit at Montefiore Medical Center—the country's first specialized headache clinic—he was also influential in neurology, having served as president of the American Board of Psychiatry and Neurology and as trustee and fellow of the American Academy of Neurology. But, according to insider accounts, Friedman had little respect for AASH, which he felt lacked credentialed leaders.[29] Graham and Diamond were both prominent physicians, but they were internists, not neurologists. Friedman was also appalled that the flagship journal of the organization was being edited by Lee Kudrow, an osteopath, since at that time osteopathy was not considered to have the same credibility as mainstream medicine. By 1977, however, Graham and Diamond had convinced Friedman to join. Friedman was immediately elected president of AASH, serving from 1978 to 1980, and Donald Dalessio, a neurologist, was appointed in Kudrow's place as *Headache* editor. Not coincidentally, the organization, which typically received about 20 to 30 new members a year, experienced a sudden influx of 410 new members.[30]

Not long after, several young neurologists reorganized the leadership structure of the association. They forced Diamond out of his long-term leadership position and elected a series of neurologists to official positions. According to neurologist folklore (at least a half dozen people told me this story in a hushed voice, making sure nobody else knew they were spilling the beans about how neurologists tossed aside the internists who used to run the AASH), the transformation of the AASH leadership was part of the effort to make headache medicine more "scientific." As one prominent headache specialist, a neurologist, described to me in an interview, "it was neurologists who said: 'enough is enough—we have to have representation for the scientific side, and we have been talking about the same thing over and over. Why hasn't this field grown like other fields in biomedicine, scientifically?' " But what neurologists in headache medicine recount as the process by which headache medicine was made more scientific might more accurately be described as the legitimization of the disorder through its reconstitution as a mechanism-based specific entity. The AHS remains interdisciplinary, but neurologists have made up the majority of the membership (currently about 60 percent) for many years, raising concerns among some that it might become a "single specialty society."[31] (The next most prominent specialty is pain management, which constitutes 17 percent of the membership.)[32] Even if the membership of the AHS has remained interdisciplinary, its leadership has long been composed of neurologists.

One of the new generation's first tasks was to overhaul the diagnostic criteria for migraine. In order for neurologists to identify the specific biological mechanisms causing headaches, they needed to be able to perform reliable experiments. The results of any experiments were meaningless without rigorously standardized diagnostic criteria. Indeed, an overhaul of diagnostic criteria would prove to be essential for the conduct of randomized clinical trials (RCT) on new pharmaceuticals. An ad hoc committee organized out of the National Institutes of Health (NIH) had developed the first set of criteria in 1962, but this early classification system was too vague to be useful for the kind of ambitious new research the neurologists wanted to perform.[33] For example, the 1962 criteria described migraine attacks as "commonly unilateral" and "usually associated" with nausea and vomiting. But if a migraine did not always involve these symptoms and sometimes presented with, say, bilateral pain and no nausea, researchers were given no guidance for diagnosis. As a result, researchers could not feel confident that they were uniformly enrolling patients with the same disorder. According to Danish neurologist Jes Olesen, "new research results were often dismissed with the comment 'How can you be sure that they really studied migraine?' "[34] In other words, how did they know that the object of their investigations was real?

Inspired by psychiatry's Diagnostic and Statistical Manual of Mental Disorders (DSM), Olesen set up a committee to work on what became the first International Classification of Headache Disorders (ICHD-I), published in 1988. A second edition, the ICHD-II, replaced the ICHD-I in 2004 and significantly multiplied the number of diagnoses. Like the DSM, the ICHD made headache disorders quantifiable so that a diagnosis of migraine could be determined in a step-by-step process that counted the number of objective symptoms experienced by a patient. A physician in any part of the world could now determine whether a patient's symptoms "fit" a diagnosis of migraine. As such, diagnostic criteria have made migraine "real" by transforming it into an internationally recognized assemblage of symptoms, its universality verified by replication across national borders and cultural differences. Moreover, the classification system produced a map of headache specialists' jurisdiction, staking out the symptoms for which headache specialists were responsible and ruling out those, like depression and anxiety, that were seen as comorbid with migraine rather than a constitutive part of the disorder.

A related development has been neurologists' search for some sort of visible criteria through which migraine could be diagnosed. Headache specialists argue that "the lack of any demonstrable gross pathological change or any other readily identifiable biomarker," combined with the absence of any effective treatments, "stigmatized headache sufferers, relegating migraine and other headache disorders in the minds of many to the category of psychosomatic complaint."[35] Although technologies for measuring the activity of blood vessels had been available since the 1940s, new neuroimaging techniques have enabled researchers to provide much more detailed accounts of the activity of the brain during a headache and have played key roles in transforming headache from a condition of the vascular system and the mind into a disorder of the nervous system. Although methysergide raised questions about the vascular theory of migraine in the 1960s, cerebral blood-flow imaging dealt the vascular theory of migraine a devastating blow in the 1980s by showing that in some patients the headache began while the blood flow was still decreased and before dilation. In the 1990s, researchers used new functional magnetic resonance imaging (fMRI) technologies to detect cortical spreading depression (CSD), an electrophysiological excitation of the cortex that is now thought to be the pathophysiological mechanism behind migraine aura. In another important study, researchers used positron emission tomography (PET scan) to propose the existence of a "generator" within the superior brain stem responsible for initiating migraine headaches. Neurologists hope that imaging techniques may one day prove to be a "mechanism-based" means of diagnosing different headache disorders, replacing the messy complexity of the clinical encounter. Imaging technologies that foreground the brain help fade the patient into the background.

Efforts to trace the genetics of migraine have contributed to a sense that migraine is "real." Doctors have long known that migraine runs in families, but it wasn't until the 1990s that they began seeking a genetic basis for migraine disorders. Population-based studies, some using twins, found clear evidence that migraine is, at least partly, inherited.[36] In 1996, Roel Ophoff and Gisela Terwindt located a genetic basis for familial hemiplegic migraine, a rare, autosomal dominant form of migraine with aura that is accompanied by a variety of neurological symptoms, like numbness or paralysis on one side of the body.[37] This was followed by the discovery of two additional genes causing the same diagnosis, suggesting that it is more appropriate to talk about various forms of migraine, rather than migraine as a singular entity.[38] Newer studies have located genetic regions likely to carry a mutation for migraine. Although the literature demonstrates that genetics is only one of many causes of migraine (accounting for about 61 percent of heritability), with each genetic discovery, researchers often declare that the public will finally take migraine seriously.

But perhaps the most significant development for the status of headache medicine was the emergence of effective pharmaceutical treatments for migraine. In 1991, pharmaceutical giant Glaxo (now GlaxoSmithKline) began distributing Imitrex (generic name: sumatriptan), a drug that headache specialists often describe as "revolutionary." The importance of Imitrex lay, first of all, in its efficacy. The earliest clinical trials reported that it could abort migraine in about half of those who used it and reduce pain in more than 70 percent.[39] Clinicians described the "'miraculous' and rapid disappearance of their patient's symptoms after subcutaneous injection of sumatriptan during a severe migraine attack."[40] Although Imitrex was not the first drug capable of aborting a migraine (dihydroergotamine had been available for decades), Imitrex worked faster, on more people, and was more marketable. For many people in pain, Imitrex was the first therapy that had ever aborted a migraine in process. Sumatriptan, the drug in Imitrex, is also remarkably specific. Like methysergide, it mimicked the neurotransmitter serotonin, which had complex effects on blood vessels. But unlike previous drugs, sumatriptan targeted specific serotonin receptor types (called 5-HT_{1B} and 5-HT_{1D}) located in the cranial rather than peripheral blood vessels and nerves, thereby avoiding many of the serious side effects produced by activating other 5-HT receptor sites. Its safer side effect profile made more doctors feel comfortable prescribing it to a broad patient population. It quickly became a blockbuster drug, inspiring four other major pharmaceutical companies to develop six more members of the triptan family, each a minor variant of the original.

Physicians finally had a tool in their doctor's bag that made them feel like they were helping their patients. Imitrex's creator Patrick Humphrey claimed to have "been warmly, if politely, kissed by many more women than I would have, had I not been credited with its discovery."[41] Even better, triptans meant headache specialists, like other specialists, could now treat their patients with medication instead of having to get involved in complicated discussions of individual psychology. By the same token, the drug's effectiveness meant that patients would no longer be suspected of faking their pain or bringing on their own symptoms. As Humphrey himself declared, "the discovery of sumatriptan confirmed, once and for all, that migraine truly is an organic disease and not just the figment of imagination of 'neurotic' patients."[42]

In this account of the development of Imitrex, Humphrey makes explicit the underlying assumptions of the neurobiological turn in headache medicine. For headache specialists, reducing the disorder to a specific mechanism in the brain doesn't just relieve the symptoms of migraine; it also targets the stigma associated with it by shifting responsibility for the pain away from a weak or neurotic personality toward a body over which the patient has no control. In this, headache specialists are demonstrating a phenomenon known to cognitive psychologists, namely, that attributing low causal responsibility to stigmatized behaviors reduces blame and produces more positive feelings.[43] Similarly, anthropologist Joseph Dumit has shown that psychiatric patients see PET scans of disorders such as schizophrenia and depression as powerful tools of destigmatization and legitimization, since "the diseased brain, in this case, becomes a part of a biological body that is experienced phenomenologically but is not the bearer of personhood."[44] In the same way, images of the migrainous brain promise to destigmatize and legitimate patients by separating out their pain from their personality. As technologies have foregrounded the brain, the patient appears to recede into the background. This is quite a good thing for headache specialists who have always found that the patient complicated their status within medicine: *The patients aren't causing their headaches; it's their brains.*

In migraine, of course, separating out the pain from the person means specifically separating it from women. Headache specialists repeatedly argue that migraine used to be understood as a women's disease, but that the turn to the brain proves migraine to be a gender-neutral disorder that transcends individual psychology and social environment. As former AHS president Stephen Silberstein told public radio listeners, "We used to believe that migraine was a disorder of neurotic women, whose blood vessels dilated and they couldn't face up to life. We now know that migraine is a disorder of the brain."[45] Valerie South, chief operating officer of the IHS, tells the same story: "For the past 100 years, migraine has been thought of as an imagined disorder and as only a woman's problem. . . . Physicians believed women were stressed out from taking care of children and from the lack of ability to cope, but recent research has underscored the fact that migraine is a real biological problem."[46] In other words, headache specialists exaggerate the association between migraine and women in the medical literature (since, as we saw in the last chapter, men had migraine personalities, too), while casting the framing of migraine as a "real biological problem" in opposition to the framing of migraine as a "disorder of neurotic women." The brain and gender are seen as mutually exclusive categories.[47]

This isn't to say that contemporary headache specialists ignore gender altogether; indeed, it would be difficult to ignore that three times as many women as men have migraine and that almost all of migraine patients are women. However, neuroreductionist models have enabled headache specialists to bracket gender as something not of their concern. As headache specialists see it, the brain is the fundamental cause of migraine; all else, like sex hormones that may trigger migraine, is external. For headache specialists, the brain has no sex, despite numerous and widely reported scientific studies making sweeping claims about the fundamental differences in the neurophysiology of men and women.[48] Indeed, much of the purported legitimizing power of the brain hinges on the challenge it offers to what headache specialists think of as sexist psychosomatic theories of the past. Claims that migraine is a neurobiological disease offer the chance for headache specialists to present a gender-neutral explanatory framework for migraine.

Policing the Brain

Headache specialists believe so fervently in the neurobiological paradigm that they perceive other potentially productive areas of inquiry as off-limits, leaving those who hold alternative views feeling marginalized. Nevertheless, dissenters remain. Many of those who argue vociferously against the trend toward neuroreductionism are members of a subsection of the AHS called the "Behavioral Issues" interest group, which works toward increasing the "understanding of the role of psychological, social, emotional, behavioral, and psychobiological factors in headache."[49] Its members tend to be people with doctorates (not MDs) who work on nonpharmacological, nonbiological aspects of headache. While they are active in the membership and occasionally win the right to run a symposium, they remain marginal to AHS leadership.

The small group of individuals with whom I spoke expressed great frustration with both the general direction of headache medicine and the specific leadership of the AHS. At best, they felt that the leadership of the AHS was taking the organization down the wrong clinical path, since external triggers are often easier to control than internal pathophysiological processes. They worried that neurologists and pharmaceutical dollars had co-opted the professional society. As one researcher told me in an interview:

> When you go to headache meetings, it's pretty impressive that most of the people, the "powers that be," are, you know, promoting the idea that this is receptor pathology and that there is hardly an individual attached to the headache. It sounds like there is a free-floating headache that you can treat without regard to the human being. The research that does look at individuals like patient preferences is very pharmaceutical driven. You know, it's what do people want out of a drug? And most of the psychological research is considered isolated rather than integrated with the rest of the headache research.

In other words, the complaint is that the patient disappears as the brain comes into focus.

Another headache specialist, this one an internal medicine physician, used the analogy of a smoke alarm to describe what he felt were the limitations of his colleagues' focus on pathophysiology. It was as if, he argued, a smoke alarm went off and everyone focused on "how the bell rings, how the electricity goes into the bell and what different things happen . . . when the smoke alarm goes off, [i.e.] how the smoke changes into electrical signals and then it sounds the alarm." This understanding of the process, he argued, ignores the very factors that triggered the alarm in the first place. The danger, he argued, was "if you get a powerful migraine drug that is developed by basic research and you simply give that, but not address what caused it in the first place, it can lead to more problems" (interview).

Some advocates of the psychological perspective interpret the AHS's adherence to a neurobiological model of migraine as a reaction against the (sexist) psychosomatic explanations of migraine popular in the 1960s and 1970s. As one prominent psychiatrist in the AHS put it:

> That [neurobiological] paradigm is going to be very hard to convince the others to change . . . those guys wouldn't go for that. When I started working with headaches twenty years ago, people were talking about migraines as a result of repressed anger and real psychological causes. Really. The lectures were just like that! And, maybe it's because of that history, but there's a real resistance to talking about anything but the biological. Maybe now we're at a point where we can start looking outside biological causation, but I'm not sure we're ready. . . . This group is wed to a biological paradigm. (fieldnotes)

Many of the headache specialists with whom I discussed this with agreed. Several even described ways in which the neurobiological paradigm is policed, a professional phenomenon that science studies scholars refer to as boundary-work.[50] Boundary-work, as described by sociologist Thomas Gieryn, is a process through which groups of scientists legitimate their practices by denouncing and distancing themselves from others. In headache medicine, boundary-work positions the neurobiological paradigm as objective science in opposition to the gendered subjectivities of a psychosomatic paradigm; nonbiological explanations for migraine are discursively coupled to a delegitimizing, stigmatizing, and feminized discourse. As a result, there exists a real fear in the broader community of headache specialists of allowing any psychological discourse to enter into the research arena, lest the headache community revisit the sexism and victim-blaming of psychosomatic medicine.

Although headache specialists defended this practice as coming from a well-intentioned place, they suspected that gatekeeping occasionally squelched competing perspectives that might better explain some of their patients' problems. In the following interview excerpt, one such headache specialist—a leader in the field—explained the problem to me as one that is entrenched in fears that psychosomatic theories of headache merely gloss over a real biological problem: "Before medicine can explain what's going on, you know, especially if they are conditions that are more common in women, they tend to be attributed to psychiatric or psychological factors or sometimes the implication is that they are excuses for not wanting to function. You know, the old joke about 'not tonight I have a headache.' And then as we become, as we understand more about the physiologic underpinnings, the diseases are legitimized in a way, and the stigma is removed, and it seems that that is happening with headache." She is well aware that women might suffer from physicians who glibly categorize their pain as psychological when, in fact, a better biological explanation exists. But then she worries that this paradigm blinds the profession to alternate theories of causation, relevant to some of her patients:

> I think that it's possible to go overboard. We still do see . . . patients where I'm quite convinced that the underlying explanation for their headache complaint is psychiatric and that it's not a combination of someone who has two disorders which is most often the case. You know most often you have someone who has depression and has migraine and it's not that case that one is causing the other; they're both conditions that the patient has. But, we do see patients who fairly clearly have headache as an example of conversion symptom. It's not common, at all. But I think one of the things that I notice that this wholesale adoption of the idea that headache is entirely a biologic illness has caused people to perhaps think [is] that because most of the time it's a biologically based illness, it can never be a psychiatrically based illness. And I think it can, there really do seem to be cases that have largely psychiatric underpinnings. . . . I'm actually just collecting a number of cases where it really seems very clear, having followed these patients for . . . at least over a decade, that their headaches really are psychiatrically mediated. And I don't mean to suggest that that's usually the case; I think it's all for the good that headache is being looked at as a biological illness, but what I think is a problem is that sort of closes people's minds to the idea that there might occasionally be other explanations. (interview)

I attribute the length of this headache specialist's answer to ambivalence. On the one hand, this specialist knows that medicine has a real problem with attributing disorders with low disease specificity to the psyche, especially when those disorders happen to women. Indeed, she expresses a genuine desire to attribute migraine to biological factors as a means of alleviating headache patients from any responsibility for their pain. On the other hand, she has experience with patients who have psychiatric problems and who, in her opinion, are likely to have psychogenic pain. But she has real worries, produced through boundary-work, about verbalizing these concerns, both for her patients and for what it says about the state of her profession. She might address this by collecting and publishing a series of clinical case studies in which she argues that psychology plays a causative role in migraines—a paper that she has yet to submit for publication.

The Migraine Brain as a Gendered Brain

Ironically, the neurobiological turn in headache medicine may not in fact be able to legitimate or destigmatize migraine. In the past few years, social scientists have raised doubts about the ability of biological models to alter public opinion about contested disorders that have a mental component. Sociologist Jo Phelan, for example, has shown that attributing schizophrenia to genes actually intensifies stigma by making the stigmatized person "seem more fundamentally different than others."[51] Phelan's findings lead her to question the assumption made by attribution theorists that embodying causal responsibility for an illness reduces the stigma attached to it. Rather than separating the person from his or her pain, she finds that "genetic essentialism" actually ties the person ever more closely to the illness, since "genetic factors are increasingly viewed as the basis of an individual's identity and as strongly deterministic of behavior." Using neurobiological explanations for illnesses also offers little help. A study by sociologist Bernice Pescosolido and colleagues found that, although the public is now much more likely to attribute major depression to neurobiological causes than they were in the mid-1990s, this new causal attribution has done little to reduce the stigma associated with depression.[52]

These results are counterintuitive. Nobody expected biological explanations of disease to result in higher levels of stigmatization. The puzzle, then, is to figure out why it is that biological explanations of mental illness have had this effect. One possibility is that neurobiological explanations, so often designed to erase the person from the clinical encounter, do not ultimately protect people from responsibility for illness because, in Western culture, the brain is too closely aligned with personhood.

A close examination of medical talk about migraine reveals that the neurobiological turn in migraine has not erased the idea that migraine affects a particular *kind* of person. To the contrary, a specific kind of moral character remains embedded in new neurobiological explanations of migraine—this time in the form of what is sometimes called "the migraine brain." The migraine brain, according to Carolyn Bernstein, founder and director of the Women's Headache Center at Cambridge Health Alliance and Elaine McArdle, coauthors of a book titled *The Migraine Brain*, refers to the highly sensitive, overreactive neurological system of the person with migraine: "The average person's brain doesn't react too dramatically to minor irritations or interference. . . . That's generally not true for people prone to migraine. [The migraine] brain is as high-maintenance as they come. Like a thoroughbred racehorse or diva, it's hypersensitive, demanding, and overly excitable. It usually insists that everything in its environment remain stable and even-keeled. It can respond angrily to anything it isn't accustomed to or doesn't like. . . . A Migraine Brain is always on alert, ready to overreact to any stimulus it finds displeasing."[53] Bernstein and McArdle argue that the migraine brain is a neurotic organ, prone to throwing temper tantrums at even the smallest environmental changes. Although migraine differs from most psychological disorders in that it is not a disorder that alters the personality, people with migraine do often act in ways that others may deem antisocial. It is typical (and recommended), for example, that people with migraine avoid anything that might trigger an attack, whether that trigger might be red wine, lack of sleep, fluorescent lighting, or wafts of perfume. As a result, a person with migraine might abstain from alcohol, leave parties early, or insist that friends forgo perfumed lotions. In 2010, a Detroit woman successfully sued her employer for failing to keep coworkers from wearing scented products that had been triggering her migraines.[54] Bernstein and McArdle argue that such people are not themselves "high-maintenance"—even if they may seem that way. Instead, it is better to think of them of being in possession of high-maintenance brains. The migraine brain, thus, serves as a neurobiological explanation for many of the same personality quirks that have always been ascribed to those with migraine—a tendency to demand that environments change to their desires, rather than a stoic ability to adjust to the changing world. Bernstein and McArdle's migraine brain displaces responsibility for this preciousness onto the brain, a move that may actually have the effect of reifying what might otherwise be a malleable feature of one's personality.

Bernstein's "migraine brain" is a popularized version of "the sensitive brain"—a metaphor used by headache specialists to explain and understand the physiology of migraine. Peter Goadsby introduced the "sensitive brain" in 2001 as part of a major effort by the AHS and the AAN to educate physicians about headache disorders. The term "sensitive brain" was meant to describe a range of findings in which people with migraine were found to have a nervous system that, in one way or another, maintained a lower threshold for change than "normal" brains. Goadsby, not oblivious to the term's potential for stigmatizing patients, joked to the large audience assembled to hear the first lecture from this collaborative educational initiative, "This is not the new-age sensitive brain. . . . This is the concept of sensory sensitivity" (fieldnotes).

He continued to explain what he meant: all brains could conceivably produce a migraine if agitated enough, but people with migraine react to much smaller irritants, like alcohol, certain foods, sleep irregularities, stress, perfumes, hormonal shifts, weather and altitude changes. Any one of these triggers might not be enough to initiate a migraine attack, but multiple triggers could build upon one another, eventually overwhelming that individual's threshold for change. This "threshold," however, varies by person and is genetically predetermined. A person with migraine, then, has inherited a brain with a lowered threshold for withstanding change that can be described as *hyperexcitable*, *sensitive*, or *overreactive*.

No matter which term is chosen, a consensus has emerged that the migraine brain is "different." Stephen Silberstein and *Headache* journal editor John Rothrock further explain this concept in a Continuing Medical Education program: "The clinical syndrome of migraine may reflect a sensitive brain. Studies have suggested that migraineurs chronically exist in a state of cortical hyperexcitability . . . that is characterized by a reduced migraine threshold."[55]

This conceptualization of the "migraine brain" has been hastened by pharmaceutical industry–funded studies that showed that antiseizure medications, especially Topamax (topirimate), could prevent some migraines. The idea thus bloomed that these drugs worked by "lowering hyperexcitability," thereby raising individual thresholds to environmental change—or, at least, this was the metaphorical understanding of how these drugs work. Since this metaphor has been put in place, headache specialists have encouraged their patients to adopt lifestyle changes (which had long been recommended for the prevention of migraine) in the name of promoting the stability of the brain. Patients are told to keep a regular sleep schedule; to avoid stressful situations, alcohol, food triggers, and smells; to limit travel; to eat regularly; and to exercise, preferably by doing yoga or walking. As Dr. Christina Peterson, medical director of the Oregon Headache Clinic, once put it to a radio audience, "those of us with migraine have very sensitive brains, and that sort of enforces a boring life."[56]

Headache specialists explicitly use the sensitive brain metaphor to destigmatize and legitimate migraine. For example, in their self-help book for people with migraine, Ian Livingstone and Donna Novak describe the sensitive brain of the person with migraine as having "enhanced sensitivity" and suggest that for people with migraine, "sensitivity to change is often misinterpreted as a character flaw or inability to cope with life." They add, "these attitudes result from not acknowledging [that] this enhanced responsiveness [comes from] the nervous system."[57] But Livingstone and Novak's statement ignores the broader problem: shifting the blame from "character" to the "brain" does not remove migraine from a person's identity. Livingstone and Novak in fact tack in the opposite direction: they are quick to point out that a sensitive brain may improve character. "Enhanced responsiveness," they argue, can make the person with migraine "more lively, aware, and sensitive." Meanwhile, according to headache specialist (and former president of the National Headache Foundation) Roger Cady, a sensitive brain can help explain the emotional tumult sometimes experienced by people with migraine: "In the same way that people born with this nervous system get migraine, they may in fact in a certain way, be more vulnerable to emotional upsets in life, be more aware of the emotional context of life and that's probably the starting point that I would offer in understanding the connection between migraine and emotional life."[58] From Cady's perspective, a sensitive brain conveys more than sensitivity in the physiological sense (i.e., having a low threshold of sensation or feeling). A sensitive brain may also denote an emotional personality trait, an increased awareness of and responsiveness to the feelings of others. Even as a sensitive brain is conditioned to experience more physical and emotional pain, he argues "there tends to be this greater understanding and awareness and sensitivity of the feelings and needs in the environment, other people in their environment, um, almost an intuitive sense, which I just think reflects sort of a lower threshold to feeling and understanding things."[59] Cady's sensitive brain is remarkably similar to eighteenth-century and Victorian notions of sensibility.

Headache specialists have hoped that the turn toward the neurobiological would bring with it a more "scientific," objective way of understanding the headache patient. By understanding migraine as a disease of the brain, they wish to destigmatize migraine and, in turn, raise the status of both the disorder and their profession. But a close reading of this turn toward the neurobiological has revealed that the new notion of a sensitive brain retains the idea that people with migraine are certain *kinds* of people. They are emotionally, as well as physiologically sensitive. They are also people who cannot tolerate much change in their lives, people who are finicky about the foods they eat, the quantity and quality of sleep that they get, and the amount of stress that they can handle. The only difference between the neurobiological configuration of migraine and the psychosomatic model of migraine that it has replaced is that these qualities have been ascribed to the biological structure of the neuron, rather than the qualia of the personality.

But for the headache specialist, this shift means everything. As Roger Cady explains, "The context in the past has always been that the emotional associations with migraine, depression, anxiety, easily startled, sort of this nervousness that people with migraine sometimes have been sort of associated with [is negative] . . . [the 'sensitive brain' puts] this in a more positive light."[60] Cady hopes that the emotional aspects of migraine might be put in a "more positive light" by simply reducing the migraine patient to his or her brain. But this reduction does not adequately separate these negative characteristics from the individual, nor does it improve the cultural meaning of migraine. Rather, neuroreduction has merely reduced much of the same cultural stereotyping so popular in the eighteenth, nineteenth, and twentieth centuries to the neuron. George Cheyne's "sensitive nervous system," which conveyed aesthetic and intellectual refinements to upper-class English women, has been reborn as the sensitive brain.[61] The "nervous temperament" is reified as neurobiological and genetic. Migraine medicine has come full circle, only this time bringing with it much more sophisticated and authoritative scientific rhetoric. Nevertheless, many people with migraine embrace the "sensitive brain" as their best hope for legitimacy. It is to their story that we now turn.

CHAPTER THREE

Embracing the Migraine Brain

Heather Zanitsch, a migraine advocate, has a story similar to most of the bloggers that I interviewed.[1] Her doctor diagnosed her with migraine at age twelve or thirteen, told her to take over-the-counter analgesics, and to rest when she had a migraine. She followed his rather unhelpful advice for years, but her condition detoriorated until eventually she was getting a migraine every day. No one took her pain seriously, which she guessed was "because I used to complain about headaches frequently." Then in 2006 her migraines took a turn for the worse. In addition to the normal symptoms, she began getting numbness and tingling in her extremities and felt clumsier than usual. A family member, perhaps reacting to the fact that their family life at the time was very difficult, told her that she needed "to stop stressing out." Heather felt undermined by this response. So she turned to the Internet to seek more information. There, she found hundreds if not thousands of stories like hers; people from all over the world had organized around migraine to share their stories and to establish migraine as a legitimate disease. Heather had tapped into a vast online discussion about migraine—a discussion that she now contributes to as a blogger and an advocate.

The comments from Heather's family member reflect the daily delegitimation that people with migraine experience in both the doctor's office and society, at large. For example, at a World Headache Alliance (WHA) conference I attended outside Rome in 2003, an invited speaker—an expert on Internet advocacy techniques, invited at great expense—broke the ice by mentioning that his sister sometimes had migraines. He then followed with a series of jokes about his surprise that a global organization for headache even existed. He said: "Headaches? Who would have thought?"

Employers, even sympathetic ones, are likely to contribute to the legitimacy deficit. At the same 2003 WHA conference, another speaker—this one an expert on migraine—admitted that when her two secretaries with migraine call out of work on account of their disorder she found herself thinking: "But it's just a migraine!" Attendees, most of whom had migraine, sat quietly and listened, but later complained privately about both speakers. As migraine advocates, they were used to being dismissed, but they couldn't quite believe the level of disrespect that they had encountered at their own conference.

The kind of delegitimation that Heather and the 2003 WHA conference attendees faced will likely be familiar to people who experience contested illnesses. As many scholars have documented, people who experience subjective symptoms that cannot be objectively confirmed by biomedicine often have their experience contested by medical professionals, employers, friends, and family.[2] They experience a kind of "double disruption" in their lives.[3] Not only does chronic illness disrupt their taken-for-granted world, but the skepticism that so often accompanies these illnesses can lead to a breakdown of the normal experience of self, leaving them feeling marginalized and alone. Since women are systematically less likely to be believed when they complain about pain, this experience is highly gendered.[4] As sociologist Kristin Barker argues, when the world refuses to acknowledge and validate suffering, people can start to question their own sanity.[5] Which is to say, persistent delegitimation—the experience of living among relentless doubt—can break down one's voice, one's sense of self, one's very identity. As a result, making sense of symptoms often includes the search for a framework through which people in pain can remake their identity in a way that both incorporates their illness and that acknowledges them as whole, rational people.

When this process nudges people toward using the Internet for help, as it did Heather Zanitsch, delegitimation can also produce communities of affinity. In this chapter, I take an in-depth look at how people in these online communities—people whose embodied experiences are profoundly shaped by the legitimacy deficit—construct migraine as a legitimate disease (versus a disorder or a condition) worthy of public attention and resources. At first glance, this attempt at medicalization seems aligned with what headache specialists are fighting for: to replace highly gendered assumptions about migraine patients with a public understanding of migraine as a neurobiological phenomenon. But closer examination reveals that online communities do more than just adopt their doctors' neurobiological paradigm. Headache advocates use social legitimacy, rather than typical tools of scientific inquiry, as a primary framework through which to evaluate different explanations of migraine. So, for example, biomedical studies are welcomed when they appear to legitimate the experience of migraine, but they are ignored, critiqued, and ridiculed if thought to undermine its legitimacy. Likewise, some advocates authorize embodied experience when it fits with the neurobiological model thought to legitimate migraine, but question this same experience when it does not. In general, online communities embrace the biomedicalization of migraine, perhaps even more than their doctors do, in the service of legitimating migraine as a socially sanctioned disease—since they extend the neurobiological paradigm beyond what biomedical evidence currently supports. They do so because they believe that the neurobiological model is capable of remaking public perceptions of their moral character.

I spent years hanging out online with people who have migraine. As part of my efforts, I even began blogging on a website called Migraine.com. These interactions have fundamentally changed my own experiences with migraine. I think differently about my symptoms now; I even experience them differently. I am certainly more open about my migraines as a result of reading and talking to people online. These insights into how online exchanges can change embodied experience are incorporated throughout this chapter—sometimes explicitly. In this chapter, more than any other, my body really acted as a fieldnote.

I begin by describing migraine on the Internet as it was in 2012, the year that I collected data for this chapter. But I quickly turn from description to an analysis of these communities' discourse; I seek to understand how these online communities collectively legitimate participants' experiences and how they develop strategies to legitimate migraine to the public and to doctors. How, for example, did community members determine that neurobiology is the appropriate way to reframe migraine? What expertise do they draw upon? What is their relationship with experts? Most crucially, how does the gendered nature of delegitimation factor into the ways that online communities recast migraine? As we shall see, members of online migraine communities' use of the neurobiological paradigm has only had limited success in removing gender from the migraine brain.

Migraine on the Internet

In large part, online communities exist in place of strong patient advocacy organizations for migraine in the United States. Indeed, the state of patient advocacy for migraine in America might be summarized with an anecdote. In 2010, after a great deal of lobbying by an influential group of headache specialists, the National Institutes of Health (NIH) held a workshop on headache research that included a small group of people representing stakeholders in headache medicine: representatives from various NIH institutes, various headache organizations, headache specialists, researchers, and patient advocates. The meeting was much anticipated; the headache research community had long wished that the NIH would devote some attention to its needs, and this was a chance to be heard. But attendees drew a blank when the NIH asked how the headache research community might foster partnerships with patient groups to increase funding, resources, and education. Although a few patient advocates were in attendance, none of them could name a strong patient-driven organization for migraine.[6] According to one source, a frustrated officer from the National Institute of Neurological Disorders and Stroke (NINDS) retorted: if people with migraine disorders have all of these needs, then why aren't they doing more to advocate for their cause?

People with migraine *are* speaking out in increasing numbers, but their voices primarily reside online. Like many other ailments, people with migraine have used the Internet to engage in a form of what anthropologist Paul Rabinow has called "biosociality"—they have formed groups around the shared embodied experience of having migraine.[7] The advent of Web 2.0, in which the Internet has become a place where people interact and collaborate with each other using social media, has been particularly useful in this regard. Blogs and electronic support groups have fostered the emergence of vocal, educated, and empowered migraine patients who have created multiple communities. Together, they form loosely connected networks of cooperation and exchange. Occasionally, these discursive efforts are parlayed into political campaigns, for example, the establishment of purple as an awareness color for migraine and other headache disorders, a video project in which individuals post migraine attacks to a website to demonstrate the disability associated with migraine, and letter-writing campaigns to politicians and media outlets. Together, these efforts constitute what sociologist Phil Brown and others call an "embodied health movement"—these online communities are highly motivated by and draw upon their members' personal experience of illness to organize to change science and policy.[8] Unfortunately, these efforts have been hampered by lack of organization; to date, campaigns have been short-lived and poorly attended. (In one effort, for example, advocates struggled to get more than ten thousand signatures for an online petition.) The tide may be turning in headache advocacy, however. In 2012, one group of online advocates formed a new patient organization called the American Headache and Migraine Association (AHMA) in collaboration with the American Headache Society (AHS). In the same year, another group, Chronic Migraine Awareness, that exists primarily on Facebook launched a website, filed for 501(c)3 status, and began to structure its online activities in the form of an organization, complete with a "Founder," a "Director of Social Media Networking," and a "Research Team."[9]

The online world of headache activism has long been fostered by a woman named Teri Robert. In 2001, Robert was a typical chronic migraine patient—highly disabled, spending five to six days every week in bed. She turned to the Internet in search of help, but was dismayed at the lack of available information. So when she noticed that the informational website About.com was advertising for a "guide" who could write on migraine, she decided to apply and become her own expert. Within a few years, Robert established herself as the go-to lay expert on migraine. She began by writing online content, describing migraine from a medical perspective, answering readers' questions about migraine medicine, and building an online community of people with migraine through About.com's electronic forums. At the same time, she sought treatment for, and received immense relief from, chronic migraine at a headache specialty clinic in Philadelphia, thus becoming a great believer in the restorative powers of headache medicine. In 2005, HarperCollins published her successful self-help book, called *Living Well with Migraine Disease and Headaches: What Your Doctor Doesn't Tell You . . . That You Need to Know*, which remains one of the top sellers in the headache genre.[10] In 2006, Robert moved to a new for-profit online company called Health Central, where, as "Lead Expert," she produces online content and moderates forums for people with migraine. From 2011 to 2014, Robert branched out further, producing content and moderating user forums for Migraine.com, a website owned by another for-profit called Health Union, LLC.[11] These corporate affiliations provide Robert with a platform, but her online hosts have little control over her editorial content. She holds the copyright to everything she writes and maintains several of her own blogs.

Robert is now, arguably, the most visible and vocal patient advocate for migraine. In March 2012, for example, the Health Central site attracted 317,000 unique visitors, accounting for 342,000 visits and 1.75 million page views.[12] In addition, Robert maintains a newsletter, which has a circulation of 230,000 readers.[13] Over 11,000 of these readers are registered as members, which gives them the ability to post questions and answers in the forums or to post blog content. Robert also has close ties to headache medicine and industry, serving on the board of two headache organizations: the American Council for Headache Education (ACHE)—a doctor-run patient education organization—and the Alliance for Headache Disorders Advocacy (AHDA)—an umbrella organization that lobbies the federal government for increased research dollars. She is regularly invited to attend large headache conferences and pharmaceutical focus groups as the "voice" of migraine patients. When the NIH held that planning meeting for migraine, they invited just one lay expert—Teri Robert. In 2012, Robert founded the AHMA.

Electronic support groups have become a centerpiece in her advocacy efforts. Several other women whom she has mentored moderate these groups. They keep forums free of spam and serve as lay experts who can provide information on the treatment and care of headache disorders. They also set the tone for forums, intervening in almost every thread. The groups, thus, are a hybrid space: they serve as a place for people to gain expertise on their condition, a system of support, and a space for advocates (the moderators in this case) and participants to collectively construct migraine as a legitimate disease. Although all are welcome to join, all of the moderators and most of the participants (as far as I can tell from the discussions) are women.[14]

Dozens of new communities organized around headache and migraine have emerged online in recent years, including a group dedicated to chronic migraine. These communities, almost all organized by women, take various forms, for example blogs, newsletters, online chat rooms, Twitter, teleconferences, and Facebook groups.[15] Like the forums, these are virtual spaces where people with migraine can connect with others who have similar experiences and outlooks, share information, and support one another. Many of these bloggers, tweeters, and leaders of Facebook groups have highly disabling headache disorders, ranging from frequent, severe episodic migraines to various types of chronic daily headache (defined as more than fifteen days of headache per month). Some bloggers are never without pain. Many of them also have other disabling conditions, like fibromyalgia, depression, anxiety, lupus, or diabetes. Some rarely leave their beds, let alone their homes. Collecting disability income is quite common. The Internet allows them to engage, connect, interact, and form friendships with others who share a similar embodied experience. They post content around the clock; the Internet compresses time and space. Ironically, this uniquely embodied mode of connectivity has been fostered by what is normally thought of as a disembodied technology.

Leaders and contributors praise these "safe harbors" as places where fellow members can commiserate with each other. These outlets provide a kind of "free space" that social movement theorists often talk about as a precursor to social mobilization. As sociologists Sara Evans and Harry Boyte put it, free spaces are places in which "people are able to learn a new self-respect, a deeper and more assertive group identity, public skills, and values of cooperation and civic virtue. Put simply, free spaces are settings between private lives and large-scale institutions where ordinary citizens can act with dignity, independence, and vision."[16]

Postings in these safe harbors offer various reports from the field, ranging from research findings that a participant has read in peer-reviewed journals, to news stories about migraine, to detailed accounts of what it is like to live with migraine. The latter includes talk about bad days, doctor's appointments that went well or poorly, medication schedules and whether to change them, strategies for living and working with migraine, issues with filing for disability, or just general venting about living in pain. Multiple forums mean that there is plenty of room for disagreement, diversity of opinion, and even fighting across groups.

These spaces nurture collective identities, in large part by providing public narratives that social actors can use to make sense of their lives.[17] Participants express their new collective identities, by wearing "awareness bracelets" constructed from purple beads or purple plastic; some have even tattooed the new chronic migraine ribbon (purple with a red stripe) on their bodies. These marks are meant to attract attention to the disease, but they also indicate an ontological narrative, telling a story of "who I am."[18] The experience of migraine becomes a central part of community members' identity, to the point that some refer to themselves as "Migraineurs," with a capital "M"—an issue to which we will return below.

Read together across many websites, these postings are more than a collection of individual stories, but instead constitute a dynamic, collaborative, and ongoing embodied health movement that allows people to collectively make sense of their illness, validate each other's experiences, define the nature of their problems, and brainstorm solutions. While only a fraction of the thousands who participate self-identify as advocates, all of those who read the posts—including countless numbers who "lurk"—can use these electronic support groups to reflect on the experience of migraine, re-create their sense of self, and reconceptualize their place in the world. Online communities are maintained and written by people whom sociologist Arthur Frank might call communicative bodies—storytellers who write about their own bodies as a way of reaching out to others.[19] Their purpose is not just confessional or educational; they aim to shape how others understand their embodied subjectivities. As embodied health movements go, these communities are discursive; people writing posts think carefully about the language that they use in communicating what migraine is, its effect on individuals, and how migraine shapes identities.[20]

Revaluing Migraine

These communities seek to change how migraine is understood in the world. But before they can alter others' view of migraine, they have to fix their own. Much of the work online involves increasing self-value by validating individuals' experiences. For members of these online communities, sharing their stories is itself an important mechanism for legitimating their experiences.

"Visit our message boards any day," Teri Robert once wrote, "and you'll find posts from people whose main problem with Migraine care is Attitude—not theirs, but that of some medical professionals, some media, and much of the general public."[21] Having taken up Robert on this rhetorical invitation, I found that she was right. A virtual sign hanging at the entry of an electronic support group for migraine reads "This is a real and painful disease. We do not choose to live this life." The sign preemptively rebuffs potential attacks against the legitimacy of participants' symptoms—attacks much like the one that Heather Zanitsch had heard from her family member.

Frustrations voiced online were both big and small, usually stemming from the disconnect between the serious damage that migraine had wrought in participants' lives and the disrespect with which it was treated in the world. Ellen Schnakenberg, an advocate who has long experienced from chronic migraine, summarized these frustrations in a blog post that appeared on Migraine.com. Called "The Migraineurs Dirty Dozen," she listed "twelve things not to say to a chronic Migraineur."[22] Her examples included a number of comments that dismiss the severity of migraine, such as "It can't hurt that bad," "You can work through it," and "You don't look sick," as well as comments that suggest that migraine is a fabrication of the psyche, for example, "If you could just lower the stress in your life," "It's all in your head," and "Get a hobby, it will take your mind off of it." She railed against those who would dismiss migraine as a "woman thing" and despaired of the conflation of migraine with headache. You cannot just "take a pill" and get over migraine, she said. Such statements and beliefs diminish migraine, undermining the symptoms that she and her fellow migraineurs experience. If only, she wrote, they could just take a pill or reduce stress and get over it, people with migraine would be happier and healthier people.

Schnakenberg's post channeled the anxieties of her readership, quickly becoming one of the most popular posts on Migraine.com and attracting over 150 comments and almost two thousand "likes" on Facebook. Most commenters enthusiastically agreed with Schnakenberg, joking that they would be rich if they got a nickel for every time that they heard similar comments. But other stories were more difficult to read. Posters explained how this disjuncture between the cultural logic of migraine and the embodied experience of migraine caused lasting damage in their lives. One after another, commenters told tales of employers, physicians, family members, and friends who diminish migraine or simply don't believe that migraine could cause the kind of disability that people incur. Individually, these comments were extraordinary. But comments just like this appear with regular frequency online: unsympathetic employers fire people because they "didn't believe" claims of illness; doctors fail to provide adequate care, treating migraine as "just a headache"; insurance companies deny much-needed (and physician-prescribed) medication; and friends and family members roll their eyes and tell people with migraine to fight harder to get through the pain.

The stories of delegitimation found on online discussion boards follow a highly gendered trajectory. Individuals speak out about or seek help for migraine, but find that instead of sympathy, their complaints are minimized and attributed to a failure in moral character. Schnakenberg's post, for example, includes several feminized insults; for example, those who would tell her that she merely needed a distraction or that dismissed her symptoms as a "woman thing." In addition to the "dirty dozen," readers plead for people to stop referring to them as a number of additional feminized insults, including baby, whiner, malingerer, pill popper, or hypochondriac. One reader, evidently scarred by so many undermining comments, warned that Schnakenberg, in sharing the article, had exposed herself to the accusation that she was merely seeking sympathy—a characteristic typically associated with needy women.

Another frequent form of delegitimation comes in the form of well-intentioned, but unwelcome, advice. Online commenters describe frequent (and usually unsolicited) suggestions from friends, family, and colleagues on how to treat migraine, ranging from "drink more water" to "take aspirin" to "meditate" or "try an elimination diet." If electronic support groups are any indication, people with severe migraine resent this advice. Not only does advice-giving presume a lack of knowledge on the part of the person in pain and diminish the severity of her problem, but unsolicited suggestions also imply that she could be doing more to ease her symptoms.

The delegitimation process weighs on people with migraine. Zanitsch, now inducted into the online community, explains the burden of stigmatizing and delegitimating labels in a blog post:

> It is . . . extremely frustrating and terribly heartbreaking to know that while I am stuck in my home, suffering, that people are thinking I am nuts, stressed out, drug-addled and unreliable as a friend or person in general. It's difficult to know that at any one time when I mumble about having a migraine that someone is thinking, "Just shut up and get over it already!" I can't even say "I have a migraine" to anyone without thinking I come across as fake and/or whiny. I don't even want to say it to anyone because it happens too much. . . . I cannot wave a magic wand and make myself suddenly feel up to doing what needs to be done for anyone because I am having a hard time taking care of myself.[23]

Other people in online communities share Zanitsch's concern that they are perceived as "nuts, stressed out, drug-addled and unreliable." People feel that having severe migraine generates an image of a fragile woman who cannot cope with life; who takes too much medication; and complains about insignificant woes. Like all stereotypes, some of this is true; Zanitsch *does* take a lot of medication and she *does* struggle to keep up with work.

Yet, she cannot will herself to be well; without broad acceptance that her diagnosis is serious enough to warrant the disability that she experiences, her "excuse" for staying home seems weak and whiny. Because of these frequently stated concerns about appearing to be "whiny," part of the ongoing conversation is about the various ways that contributors had "put on a happy face" to hide their pain. "Some of the times you can hide it, and so you're not whining all the time, you're not," as one advocate told me in an interview, " 'Oh my God, I'm dying today.' You know, you don't do that, you power through it. So nobody thinks you're really sick."

Physicians were viewed as part of the problem. Boards and blogs overflowed with stories of people whose physicians reproached them for being "Type A, overstressed" patients because they burst into tears or asked some pointed questions. Dozens of stories of emergency room doctors and nurses accusing people in pain of drug seeking were much worse. In a series of blog posts on receiving treatment in the ER, Schnakenberg wrote: "These doctors will often flat out refuse to give pain-relieving medication to a Migraine patient no matter what you do or say. When I had one of these, he stood in my doorway (I was admitted), watched me agonize for a few hours, then turned to my husband and told him 'Sometimes we just can't give them what they want.' When we checked later, I was horrified to find my records were prominently marked DRUG SEEKERS."[24]

People wrote in saying that doctors told them "to their face" that this is "just a headache, take Advil," and then sent them home. Or before doctors even ask them what is wrong, they look at their chart, see a history of migraine, and say, "I will not give you a narcotic." Often, these reactions were initiated even before those same individuals could manage to say that they did not *want* a narcotic. (Headache specialists argue that most, but not all, severe migraines can be treated without the aid of narcotics and that narcotics can worsen migraine. Likewise, many—although not all—headache patients in the ER respond to and are happy to receive nonnarcotic medication).

The narratives shared in these virtual spaces make it clear that, however many doubters they encounter, people with chronic migraine are very sick. The disability associated with severe cases of migraine extends far beyond days spent in bed. Online, people talk about the ways that migraine has rendered them housebound. Driving, for instance, can be difficult; shifting lights trigger migraines and drug side effects cause clumsiness. People with migraine stay home because they fear perfumes or other foreign smells that can make them sick, or because they are simply too tired or hurting to venture outside. Kerrie Smyres, who maintains a blog *The Daily Headache* and contributes to Migraine.com, provides a thick description of what this kind of disability means for her. She began by describing a single day:

> It took an hour for me to get up, dress (in the previous day's clothes), and put in my contacts, during which time I had [my husband] cancel my appointment because the migraine was too bad. I had to sit down several times while getting dressed, then crawled to the door so I could grip the frame to pull myself up. I walked the ten steps to the bathroom and sat on the floor to rest before putting in my contacts. I spent most of the day watching [TV], though I got up and walked around after every episode to see if I felt well enough to do something. By 5:30pm, I was able to pile the roasted vegetables in a pot and fill it with water to make the stock, but I was trembling so violently that I had to lean on the counter to hold myself up. Severe trembling is another sign that I'm in the early stages of a migraine, so I took an Amerge, pushed through what I needed to do in the kitchen and watched [more TV]. It halted the migraine pain, but I never did regain enough energy to do anything else.[25]

Despite the severe disability described here, Smyres reminds both her readers and herself, "I am not a lazy person. Chronic migraine is not an excuse for me to be a couch potato. . . . Acknowledging how long it takes to get out of bed or the devastation [*sic*] a shower unsettles me."[26] She also worries how others will perceive her, even practicing a retort that she has prepared for anyone who challenges her disabled parking permit: "I'll trade your parking place for my debilitating neurological disease."[27] But even as she repeats this line to herself, she admits that it was difficult to acknowledge that her migraines were disabling enough to require such a permit.

Stories of delegitimation are widespread and devastating. Online spaces, however, provide a venue for individuals to validate each other by demonstrating, through collective sharing, that their troubles are structural rather than individual. Issues that might in other circumstances be attributed to psychological blame are transformed into social problems (to paraphrase Robert: *Their* attitude is our problem). Online discussions of the disability caused by migraine function as a sort of consciousness-raising for those who have experienced delegitimization. Consider, for a minute, reactions to bloggers' confessional posts on the exhaustion of chronic migraine. While some commentators urged people with migraine to "put on a happy face," others resented having to perform this charade, seeing it as a kind of closet that keeps people without migraine from acknowledging its damaging effects. A different frame, so this argument goes, might valorize people with chronic migraine for working *despite* their chronic pain and for maintaining creative lives as bloggers and advocates *despite* their disability. Similarly, Smyres's musings on her mixed feelings about a disability parking permit can help change readers' expectations about how serious migraines actually are—since migraine is so rarely discussed as a disability, it may never have occurred to her readers that they could qualify for a disability permit.

Social scientists have often placed a great deal of weight on diagnosis, believing it to be the primary mechanism through which medicine acknowledges that symptoms are real. Indeed, diagnosis does allow people to access health care, disability, and other benefits of the sick role. However, these stories make clear that diagnosis is not sufficient to close the legitimacy deficit for migraine. A medical diagnosis of migraine may acknowledge patients' symptoms, even as it fails to guarantee access to the benefits reserved for the ill, since neither the general public nor the mainstream medical establishment views migraine as serious enough to warrant use of these resources.

"Migraine Is a Disease!"

Members of online migraine communities are looking for social validation, as well as medical validation. By locating others across time and space who experience the same collection of seemingly odd or random symptoms, they are able to confirm migraine's ontological status. Collaborative accounts are central to collective identity formation because they allow members to bond through affiliation. As blogger Kelly Wahle put it, connecting with an electronic support group "changed my life because I finally found people who validated my experience."[28] In turn, bloggers reach out to potential readers who are imagined to be lost in fears that their illness is imagined: "For those who live with this pain, you are not crazy, and you are not alone, though this is small comfort when the pain is at its [worst]."[29]

People with migraine have a degraded "objective self"—that is, their "taken-for-granted notions, theories and tendencies regarding [their] human bodies, brains, and kinds" have been damaged.[30] Sometimes people with migraine don't even believe their own pain. To combat this, online communities encourage people to become lay experts and learn how they are, in fact, suffering from a neurobiological disease. By transforming themselves into "neurochemical selves," in which their symptoms are understood as thoroughly neurobiological in both origin and practice, people with migraine learn how to advocate for themselves, whether dealing with physicians or others who challenge their subjective experiences.[31] Grounding their collective identity in the neurobiological paradigm lends the cultural authority and objectivity of science to what might otherwise be a medically marginalized diagnosis. Their desire to be understood as having a neurobiological disease is structured by the dictates of "biological citizenship"—in other words, they hope that by reconstituting themselves as neurobiological, people with migraine will gain full social, economic, and political inclusion.[32]

The development of lay expertise on migraine is part of the ethos of online communities. By subtitling her book on migraine "What Your Doctor Doesn't Tell You . . . That You Need To Know," Teri Robert implied that readers must become better informed about migraine to receive appropriate care from physicians. Advocates consider lay expertise to be necessary; if doctors do not have the expertise to treat migraine, then patients need to pick up the slack. Lay expertise is considered essential even when people with migraine are being treated by an expert in headache medicine. For example, blogger and advocate Diana Lee argued that, for her, an important part of becoming an informed and engaged patient was learning when to trust her embodied experience (for example, noticing that drugs were producing intolerable side effects) and "when to question the experts."[33]

In the case of contested illnesses, patients often become lay experts in order to challenge dominant scientific and medical practices.[34] But migraine differs from many of these other contested illnesses in one important way. While patients with, for example, fibromyalgia and chronic fatigue syndrome must fight the dominant epidemiological model that experts use to explain their illnesses, online migraine communities embrace the dominant biomedical model of migraine. As I discuss in the previous chapter, headache specialists argue that a neurobiological model of migraine will combat stigma and delegitimation. Members of these online communities generally appreciate and trust the work of these specialists; some even describe being "starstruck" when they finally meet particularly well-known headache specialists. Ellen Schnakenberg, for instance, describes headache specialists on her blog as "my heroes, and yours."[35] The specialists, for their part, welcome the attention, as well as the patients that come to them via advocates' referrals. But this is not to say that advocates blindly accept everything that specialists say. Rather, online communities transform biomedical information, enhancing it with their own instincts, beliefs, and personal experiences. They decide which knowledge to accept using a framework structured by the cultural politics of the legitimacy deficit.[36]

Online communities' embrace of the neurobiological paradigm extends beyond acceptance. Their members *want* migraine to be a neurobiological disease, and they take an active part in making the case that migraine *is* a neurobiological disease. Their reasons are twofold: first, neurobiological explanations resonate with their experience—migraine feels like a disease that affects the entire body; and second, neurobiological explanations seem to be politically useful, since a pathology of the brain signals that the disease is real. This second claim expects that social legitimacy will automatically follow from a biological basis of disease. These assumptions are mutually reinforcing—the neurobiological paradigm resonates with embodied experience in part because, as a society, we collectively recognize "brain explanations" as real. Neuroscience bears the objective authority of science. Moreover, as advocates disseminate neurobiological explanations for migraine, they help shape the collective's subjective experience of their illness.[37]

Indeed, the phrase "Migraine is a Disease!" is something of a slogan for online communities, appearing as a header on websites and on T-shirts, mugs, and other merchandise. For example, when I asked Nancy Harris Bonk, a migraine advocate who provides content and moderates forums for Health Central, what she would tell people who need to be educated about migraine, she responded: "Migraine is a neurological disease that affects your entire body from head to toe. For some people it is so debilitating that their whole quality of life is disrupted." Bonk's description combines the biomedical language of neurology and disability with the embodied experience of what it feels like to have a disease. As she uses it, the word "disease" captures the disability, pain, and pathology that migraine causes, but it also connotes a process that subsumes the body.

Underlying Bonk's declaration is the presumption that it is important to call migraine a neurobiological disease for advocacy purposes because it conceptually connects migraine with "real" diseases. In an interview, Heather Zanitsch explained to me why this is important: "People with migraine . . . want to be able to tell their family member or their friends, 'Look, this is just as real of a disease as Alzheimer's or Parkinson's or diabetes or asthma or any other disease that's out there and just because you can't see it doesn't mean that I don't have it.'" Many advocates, like Zanitsch, compared the disability of migraine with other diseases to help make sense of migraine's place in the cultural hierarchy of disease. In this case, migraine's comparison to Alzheimer's, Parkinson's, diabetes, and asthma—diseases that she understands to be more highly valued than migraine—is a way to draw attention to the ontological status of migraine as both real and serious and, thus, to distance migraine from being understood in highly gendered, moral terms.

As advocate Megan Oltman put it to me in an interview: "There's a whole structure of understanding of what a disease is that I think doesn't involve blaming the victim. As opposed to, 'Oh she gets these nervous headaches and she is just so fragile and unreliable.'" To emphasize this distinction, Oltman maintains a chart on her website that details what migraine "is" and what migraine "is not." This chart outlines that migraine "is" genetically based and neurological. Directly opposite, she writes that migraine "is not" "your fault." Locating migraine in the brain is believed to alleviate personal responsibility, a dynamic that advocates think is important after decades of medical practitioners telling patients that their personalities caused their pain. Identifying migraine as genetic accomplishes the same task—people cannot be blamed for migraine if they were born with it.

Distinguishing between migraine and headache is central to this legitimation strategy. Migraine advocates see this distinction as crucial for changing public attitudes toward migraine. Author Betsy Blondin explained it me this way: "The 'group attitude' toward people with migraine . . . [is] the old stuff that you and I have heard for years, 'Just a bad headache.' You know, 'Why can't you make yourself better?'" The worry, in other words, is that conflating migraine with headache means that it will be understood to be a regular ache and pain—and, if migraine is a regular ache and pain, then there is something wrong with those who succumb to it.

A genetically based, neurobiological model is the key, advocates believe, to distinguishing between the two. As Teri Robert explained to me in an interview: "Migraine actually is not a headache. Migraine is a genetic, neurological disease and Migraine attack or a Migraine episode is a flare-up of that disease and if there is a headache, that is only one symptom. In fact, a lot of people have Migraine with no headache at all. But in fact, it's a genetic neurological disease, it can be totally debilitating, it increases your risk of heart attack, it increases risk of stroke, but it is not a headache." Robert also insists that people refrain from using the term "headache" or even "migraine headache" in reference to their symptoms unless they specifically refer to pain as a symptom. Migraine, she points out, has been associated with brain infarcts (areas of brain tissue that have died because of decreased blood supply) and white brain lesions (altered areas of the brain of uncertain significance). Some studies have recently shown that the number of these infarcts and lesions increases when migraine is severe, suggesting that migraine may be understood as a progressive disease in some people.[38] Robert evokes these studies to provide additional evidence that migraine ought to be considered a neurobiological disease.

These exchanges make clear the enthusiasm that advocates have for the biomedical paradigm of migraine as a neurobiological phenomenon. This enthusiasm is so powerful, in fact, that advocates end up extending the biomedical paradigm for migraine beyond what many headache specialists feel biomedical evidence can sustain. For example, the best epidemiological and genetic evidence has found that migraine, like most diseases, is caused by a complex interaction between genetics and environment, of which only a portion (albeit a large portion) can be attributed to inheritance.[39] And despite widespread acceptance among headache specialists that migraine is neurobiological, doctors have yet to reach consensus on whether migraine is a disease, a disorder, or a condition.[40] (Most professional organizations refer to migraine as a disorder—terminology that suggests less certainty about the pathophysiology of migraine. Another concern is that "disease" seems like an inappropriate label for those who only occasionally have a migraine.) Online communities have, however, an advantage over headache specialists; unlike doctors who have a professional obligation to choose the language that best describes epidemiological and biomedical evidence, people with migraine bring an embodied epistemology to discussions of migraine, filtering biomedical knowledge through their personal, lived experience. The biomedical knowledge that most resonates with them—that "feels right"—does so in large part because it speaks to their experience of delegitimation. "Disease" serves multiple purposes: it appears to have scientific backing, it "fits" with a bodily experience of progressive debilitation that so often accompanies migraine, and it seems like a useful rhetorical frame that can draw attention to the severity of migraine.

This disease frame is then used to change cultural meanings of migraine. One of the most contested aspects of the disease frame involves whether or not migraine is fatal. Advocates argue that it is, drawing on evidence associating migraine with stroke and suicide. They cite, for example, biomedical studies that have found that one subset of migraine—migraine with aura, which accounts for about 30 percent of migraine—more than doubles one's risk for a stroke, although the mechanism by which it does so is not clear.[41] This increase only conveys a small absolute risk to individuals; most headache specialists do not think of migraine as a fatal disease. However, fears of a stroke resonate with online communities, whose members are regularly reminded by advocates about the dangers of migraine.

To punctuate the urgency of these situations, advocates tell cautionary tales of those who ignored head pain only to discover they were having a stroke. Teri Robert, for example, often tells the story of a young woman named Abi who, in 2001, wrote in a chat room that she had a three-day migraine.[42] Robert pleaded with her to seek care in an emergency room, but Abi said that she couldn't ask her parents as they had already accused her of faking her migraines as a way of "acting out" and demanding attention. Abi's migraine continued and, three days later, she had a stroke. Robert, then in touch with Abi's boyfriend, was hopeful that the worst was over. But several weeks later, Abi had another migraine, which led to another stroke that killed her. It only takes a few stories like this one to convince everyone in the community that the risks associated with migraine are immediate and mortal. Abi's story is especially tragic because it is linked with the delegitimation process that binds the community together. Biomedical evidence, thus, is amplified by experiential evidence set forth in the community.

In many ways, the threat of a stroke, however remote, is consonant with the devastation produced by migraine symptoms.[43] As people often write, the pain of a migraine can make them wish for death—and, indeed, suicide is a constant threat reported by those who congregate online. Biomedical research has in fact demonstrated an increased risk of suicide among those with migraine; a recent study by a group of epidemiologists and headache specialists found that people with migraine are 4.43 times more likely to attempt suicide than those with no history of severe headache—an increased rate that they argue can be attributed to the severity of pain associated with migraine.[44] But online communities have not needed this research to legitimate their experience; nor do advocates necessarily believe that these figures are particularly accurate. In one especially moving post, a mother wrote about the loss of her son to suicide after years of struggling with chronic migraine. She attributed the loss of his life to his physicians' failure to help him cope with constant pain: "My son's words to his doc were 'please help me; I do not want to die'; that was three years ago, and my son did indeed die as his doc gave up and told him he 'needed to learn how to live in pain'—and for three years he was somehow able to do this impossible feat while in 24/7 pain." Dozens of commenters responded to this post, with many describing their own attempts at suicide, denouncing those who "belittle" their disability as "just a headache." More recently, a woman who frequented a Facebook support group for those with chronic migraine committed suicide. The group immediately began to circulate her name and picture to demonstrate the severity of chronic migraine.

Posts on attempted suicide happen frequently enough that, when I asked Ellen Schnakenberg to comment on what the biggest misconception about migraine was, she responded: "Right now, the one that hits me the most is you hear people say, 'Well pain never killed anybody.' Yet Migraineurs do die of migrainous strokes, suicide, medical mistakes, and accidents. . . . We just had a suicide in the community just about a week and a half ago, again. It happens way more frequently than, I think, even the physicians are aware of." Participants in these online communities are steeped in a daily conversation in which participants regularly post stories of disability that has reached tragic proportions: they share their thoughts of suicide and, sometimes, their attempts to kill themselves; they write of accidents they had because of migraine; they express frustration at their inability to drive, since they fear a migraine attack will render them incapacitated on the road; and they pass along tales of migraine that led to strokes. This environment does more than collectively legitimate their symptoms; in conjunction with select biomedical evidence, it enables them to present migraine as a serious disease that can cause fatalities.

Rhetorical Interventions in Legitimating Migraine

As perhaps the most visible migraine advocate, Robert is aware that broad acceptance of migraine as a serious disease will require action beyond online communities. She therefore advocates a number of rhetorical interventions that target the language that people use to talk about migraine. The most striking of these interventions is Robert's commitment to always capitalize migraine, referring to it as "Migraine disease." By capitalizing migraine—a grammatical style typically reserved for diseases named after people—Robert hopes to signal how important she believes migraine to be. The capital *M* signifies the suffering, pain, and disability that she moderates daily in online communities. Ellen Schnakenberg, who writes about her and her readers as "Migraineurs," capitalizes migraine because "it represents an entire population of people who are suffering. I consciously *think* about all of my **M**igraine friends when I hit the button on my computer that capitalizes the **M**."[45]

Robert likewise argues that individual migraines ought to be referred to as "Migraine attacks" to promote an understanding of migraine as a chronic disease that an individual has all of the time—not just when symptoms crop up. Along with her admonition that people with migraine not refer to "headaches," these changes encourage people with migraine to think of migraine as a permanent feature of their physiology that affects their whole body rather than an episodic phenomenon that primarily affects their head.

Robert has also introduced another rhetorical intervention—this one on the topic of triggers—which is more controversial within online communities. Robert insists that stress is *not* a trigger of migraine, but an "exacerbating factor" and that it be discussed using that language. (Under no circumstance would she or any other advocate allow for stress—or any other trigger—to be discussed as a "cause" of migraine, since they argue that the only "cause" of migraine is an inherited dysfunction of the brain.) Triggers are "precipitating factors," which are thought to initiate a series of events in the brain that lead to migraine symptoms. An exacerbating factor, Robert explains, is different. It "makes Migraineurs more susceptible to their triggers just as stress makes anyone more susceptible to the virus that brings on the common cold."[46] She draws some of her evidence from headache specialists, arguing that the International Headache Society (IHS), a professional headache organization for headache specialists, has taken a stand on this issue, categorizing stress as an exacerbating factor. But she also draws on embodied experience. She argues that careful monitoring of her own migraines revealed that it wasn't stressful situations that gave rise to increased migraine attacks, but rather the behaviors that she engaged in when she was stressed, for example, not sleeping enough, crying, or missing meals. She argues that reevaluating the relationship between stress and migraine may enable individuals to identify and manage more triggers and, hence, have more control over their migraines during stressful periods.

Robert has a well-thought-out biological rationale for reframing the role of stress in migraine. Having said that, her insistence that stress be categorized this way is informed by the cultural politics of the legitimacy deficit. Calling stress an exacerbating factor rather than a trigger makes it possible for her to claim that it is "a myth that people with Migraines can't handle stressful situations or high-stress jobs."[47] Another advocate, who was more forthright about the political problems inherent in conceptualizing stress as a trigger, told me that it was "dangerous" to talk about stress as a trigger, since there is "the perception that Migraineurs are so fragile emotionally, they can't handle stress, they don't get jobs, they don't get promotions, they don't get treated well socially in life, it causes a great social burden, a psychological burden because of the misperception that they are socially weak because of this disease." A number of people online shared this sentiment, posting fears that doctors use "stress" as an excuse to not treat patients with migraine or to engage in a "blame the victim" mentality.

Despite the potential political advantages of distancing stress from their disease, many people writing blog posts either rejected this framing or struggled to align their embodied experience of migraine with the rhetorical framing of stress as an exacerbating factor rather than a trigger. For example, Missy Morgan, a blogger on Health Central, often wrote about the difficulty she had in making sense of how stress, anxiety, and her overall mental state contributed to migraine. On one hand, she finds Robert's framing of stress useful as a way to close the legitimacy deficit: "I was just reading today how stress is considered by some a Migraine trigger and by others an exacerbating factor. Teri Robert explains it this way: 'Stress doesn't trigger Migraines, but it does make us more susceptible to our triggers.' For the past three plus years, I have listened to people tell me to relax, take a hot bath, [chill] out. Well, I've tried that, and I still have pain in my head every day."[48] But as she reflects on her experience with migraine, she remembers that if she: "got upset my head would hurt almost immediately. . . . So I am learning that stress DOES affect my Migraines. I personally don't believe it is the only trigger of my Migraines. I've been on vacations that were relaxing, and I still had Migraines. I can't 'make' them go away."[49] Robert's framing of stress as an exacerbating factor simply does not resonate with Morgan's embodied experience. Yet Morgan's insistence that stress contributes to her migraines leaves her in a difficult position. If stress can trigger migraine, then who is to say that psyche isn't an important factor in the onset of the disease? And if psyche is important, then do individuals become responsible for their pain and suffering? Morgan attempts to reconcile this tension by pointing out that she "can't 'make' them go away."

Morgan's blog post also reveals the way that these new epistemological models can act as a potent framework in the restructuring of collective illness experience. Although Morgan ultimately rejects the "stress frame," in favor of the disease frame, moderators and advocates quickly teach newcomers how to interpret their embodied experience within this neurobiological framework. Through iterative discussions, newcomers learn that migraine is a disease that is constituted by multiple symptoms aside from pain. Communities draw on a combination of medical information and embodied experience to construct long lists of symptoms that a person with migraine may experience, including irritability; depression; euphoria; fatigue; yawning; cravings; dizziness; auditory, olfactory, or visual hallucinations; impaired speech, concentration problems; hypersensitivity; tingling; numbness; increased urination; suicidal ideation; and allodynia (or skin soreness). Kerrie Smyres posted an excerpt of a medical book's sixty-six potential symptoms of migraine to make the point that "you're not crazy, losing your mind or faking it."[50] This post—and many others like it—encourages broad adherence to a disease paradigm that allows readers to arrange a wide array of symptoms, including mental disturbances like "unrealization" and "suicidal ideation," into migraine as a body-wide conceptual scheme.

Similarly, moderators on Health Central's forums encourage newcomers to reinterpret their migraines as a progressive disease. In one typical forum exchange, for example, a newcomer writes in with a question about her medication. Her doctor has prescribed her a medication called Toradol for her occasional migraines. After some discussion about whether Toradol is an appropriate choice for managing episodic migraine, advocate Nancy Harris Bonk asks the original poster how many migraines she is getting, suggesting that preventive medication is appropriate since "there's growing evidence that Migraine is a progressive brain disease." She cites a "recent study [showing] that Migraines can cause brain damage, and that people with three or more Migraines a month are more susceptible to this damage" and refers the poster to an online document that Robert created called "Is Migraine a Progressive Brain Disease? Yes, Migraines Can Cause Brain Damage." The exchange is typical in that Bonk uses a generic question as leverage for reorienting the original poster's framework for understanding her migraines. The exchange translates biomedical evidence (research on infarcts and white lesions) into an online claim about the severity of migraine by describing these brain changes as "brain damage."

These new understandings of migraine can then be put to use in challenging public and, occasionally, medical understandings of migraine. It is in these moments that online communities come closest to engaging in a critique of existing medical knowledge or practice. When, for example, Schnakenberg had the opportunity to engage in a dialogue with an emergency room physician on Migraine.com, she critiqued emergency departments for not acknowledging "that Migraine can be a life-threatening condition—however rare." (The ER doctor encouraged readers to inform ER doctors if their migraine was worse than normal, but denied that migraines could be fatal, emphasizing that "migraine is almost never a life-threatening event.")[51]

Schnakenberg's public confrontation of a physician was somewhat unusual. More typically, online communities use embodied knowledge to challenge lay understandings of migraine. Robert, for example, suggests that readers keep information about migraine in their handbags to distribute to anyone who needs a little educating. She has created a letter titled "Understanding Migraine Disease and Migraineurs" that anyone can download, print, and distribute. The letter includes ten bulleted facts about migraine, including the following:

- Migraines are **NOT** headaches. Migraine is a **neurological disease**, similar in some ways to Epilepsy.
- Migraine Disease is **NOT** a psychological disorder. The Disease and all its symptoms are neurological in origin and very, very real. Migraineurs are not neurotic, lazy, "high-strung," overly emotional, or faking. They are in very real pain and physical distress.
- **A Migraine attack can actually be fatal.** An otherwise healthy twenty-one-year-old member of our community died of a Migrainous Stroke in November 2001.[52]

Other bloggers encourage similar behavior. Jamie Valendy of the blog *Chronic Migraine Warrior* suggests this elevator speech for those who are unfamiliar with migraine: "Migraine is a neurological disease that affects more than 30 million Americans. Despite the number of people it affects, Migraine is often misunderstood, misdiagnosed, & greatly lacks funding for research. Migraines vary in intensity, duration, & frequency; & are more than just a headache: the accompanying symptoms, such as sensitivities to light and sound, nausea, visual changes, can be just as, or more, disabling than the headache pain."[53] Online communities help people engage in this kind of intervention by providing community, support, and knowledge. As another blogger put it, "It has helped me tremendously to 'join' the rest of US [migraine online communities], and I feel like I have *migraine-backing* now whenever I quote a stat or talk about a trigger."[54]

And this is exactly what Heather Zanitsch did. She went online, found others like herself, educated herself on migraine, and then used her newfound knowledge to explain to her family member, "The things that I'm reading and the research and everything is saying that a migraine is not just a headache; it's this complex neurological disorder and that sometimes people have to see a headache specialist in order to get it under control." Online communities offered Heather a new illness identity, which allowed her to challenge her family member and seek better health care.

Heather's new identity incorporates a new vision of herself as someone who has a serious pathology of the brain. Advocates are working to promote this understanding of migraine, in opposition to the commonsense notion that migraine is a phenomenon within the range of normal experience. This political move is a striking, in large part because it is a deviation from the disability rights movement, which insists that disability is normal and that social, political, and economic structures must change to accommodate and include those with disabilities. As we will see, constructing migraine as a pathology of the brain has consequences.

Embracing the Migraine Brain

The neurobiological paradigm has attractive features beyond offering a salve to the legitimacy deficit. It is also "good to think with." Without it, the migraine experience can be fickle, slippery, and difficult to grasp. Not only is pain invisible, but as a "whole-body experience," migraine is disconcertingly complex. For years, I was convinced that my pillow gave me migraines. It made sense to me; I woke up every day with a painful crick in my neck and a migraine began shortly after. Migraine is a trickster in other ways, too. One day, stress can seem to bring on a migraine and then, a week later, a highly stressful situation might keep a migraine at bay. One might experience difficulty concentrating, but never know if this is a symptom of migraine, a side effect of medication, or a normal part of one's constitution. Fatigue can be a precursor to a migraine, a side effect of migraine medications, an outcome of a migraine, or completely unrelated to the migraine. As complicated as neuroscience is, the brain offers a tangible object through which symptoms can be understood and, perhaps, manipulated. Envisioning migraine as a brain disease enables people to reinterpret their pain through nerve pathways that travel from neck to head to sinuses; to theorize how stress acts as a "trigger," exacerbating factor, or suppressor of a "sensitive" nervous system; to conceptualize mental confusion in terms of neurotransmitters; or to categorize fatigue as a symptom of aura, part and parcel of a unique migraine attack. The neurobiological paradigm is seductive.

The brain also provides a model that enables people with migraine to compartmentalize their migraine attacks, allowing them to distance themselves from the phenomenon that causes them so much pain. The brain allows them to separate the migraine from their self. Take, for example, Teri Robert's advice to those who say that they feel "useless" or "defeated" by their migraines: "One thing I've learned it that when I feel these emotions during a Migraine attack, I need to remind myself that the Migraine attack is causing fluctuations in the levels of neurotransmitters such as serotonin and norepinephrine in my brain, and those fluctuations wreak havoc with our emotions. So I know I tend to feel these even more strongly during a Migraine. I remind myself that the Migraine is messing with my brain, and I'll feel better emotionally as well as physically when it's over."[55]

Robert's formulation offers her readers permission to split their minds in two, relegating one part—a part that is beyond rational control—to the body and keeping one part (the part which can be "reminded") to oneself. This conceptual shift serves to reinstate a useful Cartesian antagonism between mind and body that allows individuals to detach themselves from the pain that they are experiencing. Perhaps more importantly, it displaces agency from the person who has migraine, granting it instead to the migraine that is "messing" with the brain.

For advocates, the most important outcome of framing migraine as a genetic neurobiological disease may be the presumed ability of this rhetorical shift to alleviate personal responsibility for migraine. Take, for example, a blog post written by Megan Oltman as a hypothetical response to someone who might accuse her that her migraines are "in her head": "Migraines *are* in our heads—and in other parts of our bodies as well. They are a series of rapid firings of a bunch of overexcited neurons—in our brains, which happen to be in our heads. . . . So what? Just because something is taking place inside our head doesn't mean we have control over it."[56] Here, Oltman depends on the neurobiological paradigm to flatten mind into body. Saying that migraine is "in our heads," she points out, does not necessarily mean that migraine is "in our minds." But Oltman makes an interesting move—for her, migraine isn't just "messing" with her brain; migraine *is* her brain, yet it acts autonomously, independent of her will.[57]

Oltman isn't alone; people in online communities are, with increasing frequency, talking about their brains as entities that exist separately from themselves. For example, when migraine blogger Janet Geddis facetiously complains about how "I'm going to have to get the rain to stop coming and going as it does so that the barometric pressure doesn't wreak havoc on my brain," she separates "I" from her brain, despite the fact that in other contexts, she might actually locate "I" *in* her brain.[58] Similarly, Diana Lee points out in a post that it is important to monitor and regulate triggers because "Migraine brains hate almost nothing more than an interruption of their regular routines."[59] Which is to say, individuals with migraine might very much enjoy spontaneity or a glass of red wine; however, their migraine brain, which is understood to be a separate entity that a person must cohabitate with, will not tolerate it. Blogger Pamela Curtis writes that she engages in a similar practice: a neurobiological reading of migraine, she says, allows her to practice "detachment" and remember that "feelings are not fact" and that one can "measure the situation against reality and see if things check out" or if it is just a "brain malfunction."[60]

Talking about the brain as a separate entity from oneself is a way of granting distance from one's disability. It's a tendency that I understand, since I also do this; for example, in one interview transcript, I told an advocate about a particularly onerous course of treatment I undertook, which I described as an effort to "try to get my brain back on track." I like granting my brain agency outside of myself. When I have a lot of migraines, it certainly feels like my head has been taken over by an unruly entity. By thinking of this entity as a tangible object that is separate from me, I feel like I can assert some control over it. My self becomes flexible and manipulable; cellular and molecular explanations for migraine open the possibility that I can intervene and "fix" my brain in a rational manner. It allows me to detach myself from a debilitating problem that often feels too much a part of myself. Talking about my brain as a separate object might buy me more leverage with friends, family, and employers. I can explain that it isn't *me* who needs relief from required duties, but my broken brain.

This logic, however, presents an interesting dilemma. Biological explanations of illnesses of the brain do not insulate the person from responsibility for that illness in the same way that disorders of other organs might. This is because in Western countries, the brain has become the organ of personhood. As Dumit explains, with brain disorders, it is quite difficult for patients to stop with the calculation that their disorder is biological and therefore not *their* fault, since in a basic sense *they are* their brain. The separation between "I" and "my brain" is slippery and difficult to maintain. In the case of migraine, this separation requires that individuals sustain two different personalities—one that they use to define themselves and one that they use to describe their brains. I, for example, think of myself as an easygoing person, who happens to share a headspace with a difficult-to-manage brain. But at what point do the needs of my brain (for sleep, for dietary restrictions, for certain kinds of lighting) bleed over to become part of my personality? Dumit has observed in the case of depression that people in this situation often develop a complex identity politics in which they begin to describe themselves as "a particular kind of person," who shares with other people a "brain-type." People with depression, for example, begin to think of themselves as having "depressed brains." In this case, the emerging consensus seems to be that people with migraine share a "migraine brain"—a master status that determines social identity and explains people's work, social, and romantic lives. Thus, the migraine brain is an emerging politicized collective illness identity.[61] Embracing the migraine brain may, however, have unintended consequences.

Consider, again, headache specialist Carolyn Bernstein and Elaine McArdle's popular book *The Migraine Brain* (see chapter 2), which many in online communities say that they have read. Bernstein opens the text by talking about how she is also a migraine sufferer dismayed by the legitimacy problems facing migraine. As she describes it, people with migraine are in possession of a "high-maintenance brain" that loathes change. Her "Migraine Brain" (which Bernstein and McArdle always capitalize) is thus a reductionist model of the migraine personality; rather than describe people with migraine as difficult, Bernstein has described the *brain* of the migraine patient as difficult. Bernstein and McArdle argue that understanding the difficult personality of the migraine brain is the first step to treating it well.

In many ways, the migraine brain is the logical extension of the neurobiological paradigm. The brain has become so important in defining migraine that the entire phenomenon—including the character of the person in pain—has been reduced to an organ that can seemingly exist outside of the body. Remarkably, Bernstein and McArdle's migraine brain ends up essentializing and reifying gendered stereotypes about people with migraine by attributing unflattering feminized characteristics to their brains.

One might have expected the mostly female members of the online communities who spend so much time trying to dodge characterizations of migraine as symptoms of a negative moral character to reject such an analysis. But such a revolt never came; Bernstein and McArdle's migraine brain sounds normal and natural to those who have come to rely on their brain as a mechanism for repairing their moral character. In just one example, Diana Lee suggested that blog readers purchase a necklace with a pink, heart-shaped brain, since "Migraineur brains are extra super sensitive." Lee can accept and embrace a neurobiological paradigm that frames her brain as weak because she has learned to separate it from her personality.

But in a culture that views the brain as the locus of personhood, there is slipperiness between the two.[62] Indeed, online communities have wholly embraced the idea that people who have migraine constitute a particular "kind" of person. To this end, I would like to linger for a moment on online community members' adoption of the headache specialists' term "migraineurs" (usually pronounced "migraine-ers"). Oliver Sacks first popularized the term "migraineur" in his book *Migraine.* Adding the French suffix -eur or the English -er usually converts verbs into nouns: the professor professes; the teacher teaches; the runner runs. But in this case, the -eur suffix creates an agent out of a noun "migraine" that previously had indicated an event rather than an action. This linguistic trick means that for all intents and purposes, the migraineur *actively* migraines—quite a paradox for an identity that purports to alleviate individuals of responsibility for their condition. The individual is not only identified with his or her disease; he or she creates it. As it happens, people writing in online communities do occasionally write about days when they are "migraining"; they have already adopted migraine as an active verb.

As I discuss above, migraine advocates already understand the value of rhetorical interventions in shaping our collective understandings of disease. Repeatedly articulating the words "I have migraine" is different than saying "I *am* a migraineur." The latter is a matter of identity and personhood and cannot be easily shorn. The disability movement has long embraced the idea of referring to "people with disability," as in "person with epilepsy" versus "epileptics." Some might argue that this language sounds stilted or awkward, but the distinction is important. "Person with migraine" distances the individual from his or her condition. The migraineur is a new invention, a new *kind* of person.

For all of its presumed benefits, the neurobiological paradigm may also have unintended consequences for organizing a more formal social movement. For decades, social scientists have explored the ways that somatic explanations for illnesses (particularly neurobiological and genetic explanations) are overly reductionist, essentialist, and individualistic. In general, sociologists fear that by drawing attention toward proximate causes of disease, like the brain, we are blinkered from seeing the way that the broader social world contributes to the production of disease. This fear is especially applicable to the neurobiological paradigm in migraine.

Advocates' urge to run every explanation of migraine "through" the brain focuses attention on ontology, that is, the question of whether or not migraine is "real." The cost, however, is a lack of attention to social context. I noticed, for example, that much like headache specialists, online communities have very little to say about how the experience of migraine might vary across race and ethnic groups or across socioeconomic status. Although some online communities discussed the socioeconomic challenges of living on disability payments, no one discussed the possibility that low socioeconomic status might actually produce migraines. No one ever talks about race. At first, I thought that the reason for silence on this issue was simply that this topic fell outside the scope of the communities' interests. But then I wrote a blog post summarizing some epidemiological research that has demonstrated that people with lower incomes are more likely to have migraine than people with higher incomes.[63] In an attempt to be provocative, I alluded to research suggesting that the causal direction between socioeconomic status and migraine depends on whether or not a person has a strong family history of migraine.[64] For the person who has a parent with migraine, it might not matter that what his or her socioeconomic circumstances are—the person is genetically "programmed" to get migraines. But low socioeconomic status might be enough to induce migraine in people who don't have a strong family history.

The response to my post was muted. However, in an interview, one advocate referred to this post and wanted me to clarify whether I believed that socioeconomic status could be a *cause* of migraine or whether I believed it could be a *trigger.* I explained to her that this is an unanswered question, but that I believe it is important to understand how environment contributes to the fundamental cause of migraine. She seemed to think that this was intriguing, but then said: "Like you can't say all that in a blog post and have people understand, because like right away I think my feeling was: Oh, then that negates the whole disease issue, and that it's not your fault. So then you get worried, 'Oh, Joanna thinks that I can control this myself.' " I understood immediately what she was telling me. Any causal framework that incorporates a social cause for migraine is immediately suspect because, at first blush, it seems to undermine the neurobiological disease paradigm that advocates have so carefully constructed. Social class is particularly suspect because, at least in America, social class is perceived to be flexible and within individual control.

I saw this phenomenon played out again in a Health Central forum where a participant wrote in to question the credibility of research that connects child abuse with incidence of migraine. The moderator incorrectly dismissed this research as "debunked." (In fact, this research, conducted by Gretchen Tietjen, won the prestigious 2011 Harold G. Wolff research award from the AHS, in part because Tietjen found a way to theorize how child abuse might alter neurobiology.) The fact is that advocates are even more wary of social and environmental theories of causation of migraine than their headache specialists. But by insisting that migraine only be understood as a neurobiological disease, separate from any social context, migraine advocates deny themselves the ability to politicize the disease.

Reframing the Objective Self

Online communities encourage people with migraine to reconfigure their objective selves, form a new collective identity grounded in neurobiology, and then use this perspective to challenge public understandings of migraine. This new neurochemical self offers people a chance to reinvent their moral character. Blogger Pamela Curtis argues for a reframing of one's identity:

> We aren't just patients, we're healers, too—healing the hearts of others like us. We're not alone in our suffering, though it may be lonely and isolating. We're diplomats, extending the welcome to others with conditions like ours. We're ed-

> ucators, informing the public of scientific, medical, and political matters. We're activists, raising awareness for people with our condition. We're researchers, spending countless hours on the Internet looking up patient information. We're project managers, administrating the near full-time job of records, medications, symptom-tracking, billing, insurance claims, etc., etc. We may be a miserable pile of pain-ridden goo, but we are at the same time, absolutely amazing.[65]

Curtis is right: online communities seek to redefine the way that people with migraine are seen, and also the way that people with migraine see themselves. But then she adds, "Our diseases may limit what we can do, but it doesn't limit who we are."

This last sentence is important because, I would argue, the introduction of the migraine brain *is* rather limiting. By reducing the patient to his or her brain, migraine patients have embraced a knowledge system that does more than simply relieve patients of the responsibility for their disorder; the "migraine brain" rearticulates many of the gendered meanings that migraine advocates have been so desperately trying to escape. Framing migraine as a genetic and neurobiological disease may establish the ontological status of migraine as real, but the framework has its limits. The migraine brain is a useful conceptual tool for those who live with the diagnosis, but it cannot prove an individual is having an attack, nor can it assure that people with migraine are understood and treated as fully rational beings who deserve medical care and resources. In other words, demonstrating that migraine exists as a phenomenon is not sufficient to make people take it seriously.

In the next chapter, we'll see this same dynamic at work within the political economy of pharmaceutical research and marketing. While the coming of relatively effective drugs to treat migraine has, in part, validated the biological basis of disease, the industry's marketing practices have reinforced, rather than combated, existing stereotypes of migraine.

CHAPTER FOUR

Gendering the Migraine Market

Consider three television advertisements for migraine treatments:

A white woman is curled up on a red sofa, face turned into the back cushions. The sofa is not in a living room, as one might expect, but in a park, and nearby, a man and two children toss a football. The camera pans to the woman and we hear a voiceover: "When you spend more days than not separated from your own life, when the only thing you can be sure of is migraines fifteen or more days of the month, you're living a 'maybe life.'" In the next scene, the woman on the sofa appears in a mall. Two women chatting walk by her. As they do, the advertisement suggests that the viewer who is living a "maybe life" might have chronic migraine and should find a headache specialist. There is no mention of a product, but the sponsoring pharmaceutical company, Allergan, and its logo, flash on the screen at the last moment.

The television camera is focused on a white woman's face. She leans into the camera and confides, "If you know migraines, you know pain. These things are for real. But you know what? So is this." The camera cuts to her hand holding a green bottle of Excedrin Migraine. The actress demurely flutters her eyes away from the camera then back, as she explains how well the medicine works on her pain and "sensitivity to light and sound." It feels intimate, like she is telling a secret to a girlfriend.

A white woman, playing with her daughter, holds a hand to her head and we hear her voiceover: "I made a promise to Janie. Her new bike had to be ready. But my migraine just wouldn't go away. That's when I knew I had to talk to my doctor about my migraines." We see her visit her doctor and then hear an explanation of how her new prescription, Imitrex, targets the "nerves and blood vessels that trigger" migraine. The camera cuts to the woman riding a bicycle with her daughter in the sunshine.

These ads promote three very different kinds of migraine medication manufactured by three different companies: Botox, which prevents migraine by weakening the muscles into which its injected; Excedrin Migraine, an over-the-counter combination of acetaminophen, aspirin, and caffeine that relieves pain; and Imitrex, a prescription triptan that aborts migraines by acting on serotonin receptors. Despite the fact that these drugs are so different from each other, the advertisements marketing these medications look and sound remarkably the same. Each presents us with a vague description of migraine as an unwelcome and painful disruption. Each also presents us with a familiar portrait of the migraine patient: a white woman, often depicted with a family or children. When in pain, she generally looks dejected, her hand pressed to her head. With the exception of the advertisement for chronic migraine, her misery is short-lived. After the medicine has been administered, the worries in her life disappear.

The shared visual language of the advertisements is particularly striking because it differs so much from the iconography used in medical discourse. The brain, the fixation of both contemporary headache specialists and migraine advocates, is curiously absent in pharmaceutical advertisements for migraine drugs. Instead, these advertisements portray fully fleshed bodies, usually women, in pain. When present at all, references to the biology of migraine are fleeting.

The pharmaceutical industry wields tremendous power to shape both medical and public perceptions of migraine. On the most basic level, the mere existence of an effective drug to treat migraine lends credence to ontological claims about the "realness" of migraine. In addition, the specificity of triptans has altered how doctors and patients conceive of migraine, shifting explanatory frameworks from the psychological to the neurobiological. But perhaps the most persuasive messaging comes from a diverse range of marketing practices. The pharmaceutical industry spends hundreds of millions of dollars marketing in direct-to-consumer (DTC) advertising and to physicians in medical journals; through materials disseminated at conventions; at company-sponsored dinners; at detailing visits by pharmaceutical representatives; and through industry-sponsored Continuing Medical Education (CME) programs. These promotional schemes have the ability, through the dissemination of widespread messages, to construct a system of representation that marks *who* the public imagines to be the typical migraine patient. In this chapter, I focus on the images portrayed in these marketing materials. The ability to shape the pictures that people hold in their heads when they think about migraine is immensely powerful.

These advertisements, it should be clear, portray the typical migraine patient as *female*. Classic work by Erving Goffman, later expanded by Susan Bordo, has given researchers tools for unpacking the representations of gender in advertisements, for instance, by foregrounding how advertisements communicate normative values like social rank, particularly via gender.[1] Although existing research on gender and advertising is a bit out of date, what exists has found that women are generally overrepresented in medical advertisements;[2] and that both men and women are portrayed as stereotypes, with men at work and women in social or domestic situations.[3] In general, men are shown as upright, rational protectors, while women are portrayed as prostrate, sexually available, childlike, or in slanted postures. Likewise, in drug advertisements, normative representation of male patients is that of a rational or mechanistic body that is experiencing some value-free failure, while the equivalent representation of female patients depicts emotive, self-obsessed, or (in the case of older women patients) even comical women.[4] Advertisements for hormone replacement therapies were even worse, using suggestive symbols to connote menopausal women as "'out-of-control', 'grotesque', 'stressed', or 'confused' and a threat to the idealized feminine."[5] While gender norms have changed somewhat in the last thirty years, advertisers continue to depict men and women using traditional gendered representations.

Pharmaceutical advertisements for migraine medications therefore pose a puzzle for the legitimation of migraine as a serious disease. On the one hand, social scientists have found that the pharmaceutical industry has an enormous amount of power to define and legitimate diagnoses and disease entities, particularly when it has new, effective drugs to offer patients suffering from ill-defined syndromes.[6] On the other, its promotions for those same drugs consistently reinscribe the condition as gendered—a critical and ongoing factor in migraine's legitimacy deficit. After a brief discussion of what, exactly, the pharmaceutical industry is selling, this chapter follows the iconic patient in DTC advertising for migraine pain, since these are the images that we are most likely to see. While one could imagine that advertisements might serve to close the legitimacy deficit by serving as evidence that migraine is a biological entity, I argue that they are more likely to exacerbate the legitimacy deficit by representing migraine as a temporary and easily treatable inconvenience experienced by white, middle-class women.

In other words, migraine medications are gendered technologies. Their production and dissemination reproduces the commonsense notion that migraine is a condition that affects a particular kind of person—a white, middle-class woman—a construction that simultaneously stigmatizes the person with migraine, while rendering invisible other people with migraine. While in some ways new pharmaceutical technologies have facilitated biological explanations for migraine and have helped moved the discourse away from "neurotic females," the analysis in this chapter suggests that many so-called outdated cultural assumptions about migraine—as an unimportant condition that only affects a particular kind of woman—remain embedded in the patchwork of images, narratives, and rhetoric produced by the pharmaceutical industry.

The Pharmaceuticalization of Headache Medicine

Pharmaceutical sales are a cornerstone of the global economy. By some estimates, worldwide pharmaceutical sales will exceed $1.1 trillion by 2014.[7] Nearly one-third of global sales transpire in the United States.[8] The pharmaceutical industry also spends an enormous amount of money promoting its products. However, exactly how much it spends is unclear. Companies, eager to present themselves as serious, research-driven entities, are careful about how they present their marketing expenditures to the public.[9] The Pharmaceutical Research and Manufacturers of America (PhRMA), an American industrial lobbying group for research-based pharmaceutical companies, estimates that the cost of promotion ran about $27.7 billion in 2004. Independent scholars have disagreed with PhRMA's figures, suggesting that the figure is more than twice this—possibly as high as $57 billion.[10]

The modern pharmaceutical industry owes its success to its ability to market treatments for an ever-growing group of diseases and conditions (even if that means that it also must create new diseases to treat). But this multinational business was built on a treatment for the ordinary headache—aspirin.[11] Aspirin, introduced to the global public in 1899, stood as a veritable revolution in medicine's ability to effectively treat illness. Prior to the late nineteenth century, not much could be done for any sick person, let alone the typical headache patient. Headache remedies focused on relaxation cures or the removal of toxins, for example, by applying a mustard bath to the feet, or by purifying the diet. But by the late nineteenth century, a burgeoning pharmaceutical industry had discovered and begun to market drugs that could effectively alleviate headache symptoms. Bayer, an early contender, entered the pharmaceutical market in 1887 with a product called phenacetin, one of the first non-opioid drugs that could alleviate pain and reduce fevers. Twelve years later, Bayer introduced aspirin, a much more effective drug.

Bayer originally marketed aspirin as an antirheumatic drug, but it soon became clear that the wonder drug had a talent for alleviating all kinds of pain—especially the pernicious headache—with few side effects. Moreover, Bayer found that it was helpful to market aspirin straight to the public—a practice denounced by so-called ethical pharmaceutical companies, who, in an attempt to distance themselves from nostrum makers, had forsworn patents and marketing directly to the public. Bayer's practice was nevertheless wildly successful and subsequently widely adopted. The public could self-treat for head pain by buying aspirin straight from the pharmacist: no need to talk to a doctor. Bayer made its tins of pills easily recognizable; everyone knew the characteristic yellow and brown design with a cross logo (still in use today).

Aspirin remains one of the best-selling drugs in the world. One need only walk through a local pharmacy to understand that drugs for head pain, which now include acetaminophen, ibuprofen, and naproxen in addition to aspirin, constitute a large segment of the industry's over-the-counter sales. Indeed, by some estimates, oral analgesics comprise the largest segment of the $16 billion over-the-counter market.[12]

Given that aspirin gave rise to the pharmaceutical industry, it is perhaps fitting that the pharmaceutical industry now serves as the primary sponsor of headache medicine. Over the last twenty years, headache medicine has become what medical sociologists refer to as *pharmaceuticalized.*[13] That is, headache disorders of all varieties are not just biological phenomena to be studied and treated, but commodified conditions, transformed into lucrative opportunities for pharmaceutical intervention. Indeed, it might be said that all of headache medicine has become a "pharmaceutical regime," as the institutions, organizations, actors, artifacts, and cognitive structures associated with headache disorders are now linked to the "the creation, production, and use of new therapeutics."[14]

The pharmaceutical industry's stronghold on headache medicine came slowly. After aspirin, many decades passed before the industry was able to produce medications effective for the majority of migraines. In 1918, drug makers purified alkaloid of ergot, a strong vasoconstrictor, from the crude form of ergot that had been in use for treatment of migraine since the nineteenth century. In 1946, Sansert also synthesized an even more refined version of an ergot medicine, dihydroergotamine (DHE), which enabled physicians to treat some migraines via injection. Sandoz produced methysergide, the first migraine preventive, in 1962, but it was rarely used for fear of side effects. (And has since been taken off the market.) The next breakthrough did not come until 1993, when Glaxo was finally able to market and sell Imitrex (sumatriptan), the first of the triptan class of drugs. By 2007, the triptan class of drugs, of which Imitrex remains the market leader, earned over $3.5 billion for its makers.

Like many of the drugs that had come before it (aspirin included), Imitrex was hailed as a super-drug for migraine. Doctors described its ability to abort a migraine in most of the people who took it as miraculous. Its relatively safe side effect profile meant that it could be widely used. Imitrex changed the migraine experience for doctors and patients alike, helped usher in the neurobiological paradigm of migraine, and aided headache doctors in their quest to legitimate their profession.

But it may be the commercial success of Imitrex that did the most to change headache medicine. Imitrex became a blockbuster drug shortly after its American release in 1992. By 1996, Imitrex was responsible for more than a billion dollars worth of sales in the United States and £698,000 in the United Kingdom, where it is marketed under the brand name Imigran.[15] Over the next decade, several pharmaceutical companies followed Glaxo into the migraine market, producing six additional "me-too" drugs and an entire class of triptans. Seeing migraine as a viable market, Bristol-Myers Squibb and Wyeth applied for and received approval to market Advil and Excedrin, their brand names for ibuprofen and a combination of aspirin, caffeine, and acetaminophen, respectively, as remedies for migraine. (See the table 4.1 for a timeline of these drugs' release.) Although none of the triptans exceeded the popularity of Imitrex on the market and Wyeth and Bristol-Myers were simply repackaging already existing drugs, the immediate success of these new drugs diversified pharmaceutical interest in headache medicine.[16]

The financial success of new pharmaceuticals that treat migraine has

TABLE 4.1 **Drugs on the migraine market**

	Drug
Approved	Generic name (brand name)
1946	Dihydroergotamine (DHE-2)
1962	Methysergide (pulled from market in 2002)
1992	Sumatriptan (Imitrex)
1992	Sumatriptan (Imitrex, Imigran) injections
1995	Sumatriptan (Imitrex, Imigran) tablets
1996	Divalproex Sodium (Depakote)
1997	Sumatriptan (Imitrex, Imigran) nasal spray
1997	Zolmitriptan (Zomig) tablets
1998	Acetaminophen, aspirin, caffeine (Excedrin Migraine)
1998	Naratriptan (Amerge, Naramig) tablets
	Rizatriptan (Maxalt) tablets and rizatriptan orally dissolvable
1998	Rizatriptan (Maxalt-MLT) tablets
2000	Ibuprofen (Advil Migraine)
2001	Almotriptan (Axert) tablets
2001	Frovatriptan (Frova) tablets
2002	Eletriptan (Relpax) tablets
2003	Zolmitriptan (Zomig) nasal spray
2004	Topiramate (Topamax)
2008	Sumatriptan and naproxen sodium (Treximet)
2009	Sumavel DosePro (Sumatriptan) needle-free delivery system
2010	OnabotulinumtoxinA (Botox)

fundamentally altered how migraine is understood, how headache medicine is practiced, and how people come to receive care for head pain. Indeed, almost everything that we know about migraine, including our basic assumptions about *who* experiences migraine, comes from research or promotions that have been funded by the pharmaceutical industry. This is because the pharmaceutical industry has become the major financial stakeholder in headache medicine. Headache specialists, if they wish to conduct funded research and become opinion leaders in the field, must, by necessity, learn to partner with industry. And industry, through its need to advertise the medications now available to treat migraine, has by default, become the largest purveyor of public messaging about headache disorders.

The development and commercial success of triptans flooded headache medicine with cash. Each new drug required its own clinical trials and publications. Even after approval, pharmaceutical companies continued to fund studies to keep their brand name in clinics and in scientific articles. The pharmaceutical industry promoted and funded headache specialists in other ways as well. They needed "opinion leaders" to speak at conferences and at CME programs on the local, national, and international levels. Headache specialists, en masse, became members of industry-organized speaker's bureaus, using these platforms to spread the word about new medications for migraine. Pharmaceutical executives saved the biggest name experts for the biggest venues, whether national or international talks at major headache conventions or major media markets. Most of the former presidents and board members of the American Headache Society (AHS), the International Headache Society (IHS), and the National Headache Foundation (NHF) served industry in these capacities. According to their own self-reports, almost all of the presidents of the AHS, IHS, and NHF since 2001 have been involved in multiple financial relationships with pharmaceutical companies. Five individual presidents (terms at the AHS and IHS last two years) listed between twenty to thirty-one conflicts of interest, each.[17] In addition, pharmaceutical-industry support has helped transform these already successful headache specialists into popular media figureheads for headache medicine. Each of these doctors has appeared dozens, if not hundreds, of times on major media outlets, speaking about new migraine treatments.

The extent to which headache research is supported by industry money in the United States is difficult to measure with accuracy, given a lack of transparency in private funding. However, a survey conducted in Europe in 2004 is instructive. It found that of €315 million spent on migraine research in Europe, only €7 million came from nonpharmaceutical sources, including €714,000 from private foundations.[18] Similar numbers are not available for private funding in the United States, but one may presume that the imbalance in funding sources is similar, given how few public organizations in the United States are willing to fund headache research. For example, the NIH, which is the largest funder of biomedical research in the world, funds migraine research at an extraordinarily low rate. In 2011, the NIH allocated $16 million to "migraine research."[19] One might presume that $16 million is not nearly enough to hold together all of headache medicine. Funding from private sources, such as the Migraine Research Foundation or the National Headache Foundation, likely does not exceed $500,000 per year. As a result, very few institutions offer a countervailing power to the messages that the pharmaceutical industry promotes about migraine.

The FDA's 1997 decision to allow drug companies to broadcast product-specific endorsements of their prescription products to consumers amplified the pharmaceuticalization of migraine. Prior to this decision, federal regulations had limited DTC advertising, allowing it only if it provided balanced information on the risks and benefits of medication. But the practical difficulties of meeting such requirements made it difficult for advertisers to promote medication on the air.[20] The FDA streamlined this requirement in a 1997 ruling, allowing that a full disclosure of risks could be met by providing a concise summary and a source for more information, for example, a toll-free number or an Internet website. Drug companies rejoiced, throwing billions into commercials for new drugs. By 2001, spending on DTC advertising had reached an estimated $2.7 billion.[21] In 1997, alone, Glaxo Wellcome spent $36.9 million on DTC advertising for Imitrex—making it the eighth most promoted drug in the United States.[22] Spending levels remained high while Imitrex was on patent. Even in 2005, just a few years before its patent expired, Imitrex remained among the leading twenty advertised drugs by DTC expenditures.[23]

But pharmaceutical marketing takes a number of forms besides the obvious print and broadcast ads that we all see. Industry marketers use a broad array of techniques to promote their products to a variety of audiences. For consumers, these practices may include unrestricted educational grants made to organizations to provide "educational" materials, the production of television specials and stand-alone special reports, collaborations with academic institutions, public awareness campaigns that are not brand specific, and philanthropic sponsorship of community awards.[24] In her exposé on drug-company practices, Marcia Angell describes the production of "stealth ads," like the videos that journalist Morley Safer of CBS's *60 Minutes* made for drug companies. The videos, as she described them, were designed to look like newscasts, but were really promotional spots written and directed by drug companies and given to local public television stations.[25] Celebrity endorsements have also become more popular. Some are explicit, like Bob Dole famously endorsing Viagra. Until 2009, pharmaceutical companies could also use a subtler strategy: paid celebrities would make mention of a particular drug on radio and television talk shows and give interviews to reporters. Rather than publicly supporting a particular drug, these celebrities would talk about their own condition and refer audiences to "informational" websites funded by their sponsors. What the audience did not know is that these celebrities received fees for this service.[26]

In addition, the pharmaceutical industry incorporates marketing into its practices from the earliest stage of product research.[27] Marketing and promotion is taken into account when thinking about everything from which drugs to develop to the design of clinical trials to the physicians (or opinion leaders) who ought to lead clinical trials to the publication schedule of research.[28] When it comes time to sell drugs to physicians, the industry sponsors professional meetings, funds talks featuring doctors or sales representatives as speakers, and pays for Phase IV clinical trials, which are generally designed for marketing purposes.[29]

The Idealized Migraine Patient

The pharmaceutical industry has an explicit financial stake in shaping how the public understands migraine; its information, tactics, metaphors, catchphrases, and images are meant to inject public discourse with a new set of meanings and symbols with which to understand migraine. What kinds of messages is the pharmaceutical industry disseminating about migraine? And what images are missing from these depictions?

I began my investigation by collecting materials at professional headache conferences, where headache specialists reported on new research, most of which was bankrolled by the pharmaceutical giants. Every conference always had a ballroom where pharmaceutical sponsors rented expensive booths to market their products. From these elaborate booths, drug representatives attracted passersby with a bewildering array of merchandise, including pens, Post-it notepads, magnets, mugs, mouse pads, clocks, watches, laser pointers, toys, backpacks, pins, posters, radios, tape players, and books. In the early years, when the pharmaceutical industry still had many migraine drugs under patent, some companies offered separate lounge areas where conference participants could check e-mail, snack, and receive "educational" materials on medications. Large companies also sponsored satellite symposia (funded by unrestricted educational grants), at which physicians could receive CME credits. In the evenings, companies held expensive receptions at local tourist attractions. I collected hundreds of promotional materials and advertisements, including newsletters, pamphlets, patient package inserts to medications, press releases, educational materials produced for physicians, and television, radio, and print advertisements. I also conducted a content analysis of images used in a discrete sample of pharmaceutical advertisements from a cross section of websites

TABLE 4.2 **List of websites analyzed**

Pharmaceutical Website	Product Name	URL
GlaxoSmithKline	Imitrex	www.migrainehelp.com
GlaxoSmithKline (educational)	Headachequiz.com	www.headachequiz.com
GlaxoSmithKline (educational)	HeadacheTest.com	www.headachetest.com
AstraZeneca	Zomig	www.zomig.com
Pfizer	Relpax	www.relpax.com
Pfizer (educational)	MigraineRelief	www.migrainerelief.com
Merck	Maxalt	www.maxalt.com
Ortho-McNeil	Axert	www.axert.com
Bristol-Myers Squibb	Excedrin	www.excedrin.com
Health Assure	MigraHealth (herbal)	www.migrahealth.com
Ortho-McNeil	Motrin	www.motrin.com
Wyeth Consumer Healthcare	Advil Migraine	www.advil.com
MigreLief	MigreLief	www.migrelief.com
Weber and Weber	Petadolex	www.migraineaid.com

Note: Websites accessed September 3, 2003

that marketed headache medicine—each of which was owned by a company that rented booths at professional headache conferences.[30] The full list of websites included in this analysis is included in table 4.2.

The average pharmaceutical advertisement for migraine medication represents the archetypical migraine patient as a middle-class, white woman. Images—which unlike the text of advertising are relatively unregulated by the FDA—are the most obvious manifestation of this phenomenon. Most pharmaceutical advertisements keep their descriptions of migraine short, and with the exception of brief mentions of menstrual migraine, these descriptions could generally apply to a man or a woman, of any race, of any income. Yet this carefully scripted text is usually accompanied by a visual depiction of a white woman. In just one example, found on a website that GlaxoSmithKline (GSK) had set up to sell Imitrex, a large image of a white woman holding her temples appears just above text describing the basics of migraine. The headline, "Understanding Migraine," promises an explanation for migraine:

> **Understanding Migraine**
>
> **A migraine is not just a headache.** Although moderate to severe head pain is the most common symptom, there are usually other symptoms that help diagnose frequent bad headaches as a migraine. It is important for you to understand and

recognize these symptoms in order to help your doctor diagnose your headache and provide you with proper treatment.

—www.migrainehelp.com[31]

The text says nothing about the epidemiology of migraine, but the image suggests what a person with migraine might look like. This visual cue is of particular importance, given that the text provides almost no explanation of what migraine is or who gets it, beyond defining migraine as "not just a headache." Readers would have to click further into the website to learn more details about the symptoms of migraine. This advertisement is not really about "understanding migraine," but about encouraging readers to see a doctor. This format, in which the visual arrangement takes precedent over information, is part of a common trend in contemporary advertisements, many of which make little mention of the product that they advertise. Instead, advertisements now leave viewers to infer meaning from the look of the people in the ad.

This format was consistent across all pharmaceutical advertisements for migraine. In 2003—a year when all triptans were under patent and advertising for consumers was fierce—I sampled the contents of fourteen drug websites. Through a process outlined in the appendix, I downloaded the images on each of these sites and coded them for a number of features, including gender, race, setting, and pain status. Of the eighty-six images posted on these sites, seventy-nine (85 percent) portrayed a layperson with migraine. Of these, fifty-five (70 percent) had a female as the primary figure(s); four (5 percent) featured both men and women; five (6 percent) featured a heterosexual romantic couple; and fifteen (19 percent) had a male as the primary figure. Because representations of women with migraine dominate these images, pictures that portray both men and women read as though the woman in the image is the one who has the migraine. (One would never see such an image alone—they were always on websites surrounded by pictures of other women.) But these figures inflate the number of men one is likely to see in migraine advertisements. Of the fifteen pictures of men, five depicted the same man in different postures on a single website. Only ten different men are depicted as migraine patients across all fourteen websites. If I were to count these images as one, then men account for only 13.4 percent of these representations.

Both patients and health care providers were usually portrayed as white and middle class. The vast majority (81 percent) of patients depicted were white. The race of people presented in an additional six images (7.5 percent) was unclear, as each bore some subtle ethnic markers (e.g., an olive tone to the skin or features suggesting mixed race). Only four (5 percent) were clearly black. Class was more difficult to discern, though the vast majority of patients bore markers of affluence, for example, expensive-looking clothes or styled hair. With only three exceptions (i.e., an image of a worker wearing a flannel-checked shirt and a hard hat), workers were portrayed as holding white-collar jobs where they sat behind computers and wore business attire.

What were the men and women in these images doing? In only about 20 percent of the cases were they shown exhibiting pain. More typically, they were *not* in pain and *not* disabled, but rather in normal life situations, perhaps in what advertisers hoped would appear to be an "after" shot, as in "after the medication took effect." Migraine is rarely presented as a disabling disease, but as a condition easily conquered with a pill. These active, engaged, and seemingly healthy individuals were presented in gender normative scenarios, conforming to gender stereotypes.[32] For example, men were significantly (at $p<.01$) more often represented in work settings (40 percent) than women (12.7 percent). Women were as likely to be shown with children (12.7 percent), as they were to be shown at work. No men were portrayed as caretakers of children. There were, however, occasional gender transgressions in these advertisements. The website for almotriptan (Axert) portrayed a black female physician caring for a white male patient. Another advertisement, posted on eletriptan's (Relpax) educational website, depicted two women speaking at work, where one appeared to be in a position of authority. These examples reflect a changing workplace where women and minorities play an increasingly important role. But these representations are rare. On GSK's website, for example, three images portray male physicians, two of whom are speaking to female patients who appear smaller and shorter than their physicians. As Goffman suggested, such differences in size and perspective connote the "social weight of power, authority, and rank."[33]

The gendered portrayal of migraine was further exacerbated by the use and placement of male images. Although the home pages of the drugs' websites prominently displayed images of women, images of men were so deeply buried in internal pages that readers might never find them. This was true even in the rare case where the text referred to men with migraine. The home page and most of the links on a Pfizer website for Relpax, for example, offered a stereotyped vision of migraine as a women's condition. The reader diligent enough to read the entire website, however, might stumble upon two pages devoted to men. One of these pages displayed a picture of a man next to text that suggested that representation of migraine as a women's disease might be responsible for the significant underdiagnosis and undertreatment of men with migraine: "Due to a misperception that people have about migraine being a woman's disease, many men may find it difficult to ask for help."[34] The second image of a man accompanied text that read "Once thought of as strictly a woman's disease, migraine affects a substantial number of men. In fact, 1 out of every 3 migraine sufferers on the job is a man."[35]

The people portrayed as having migraine in pharmaceutical advertisements do not adequately represent the population that epidemiologists think is most likely to get migraine. Epidemiological estimates suggest that women are nearly three times more likely to have migraine than men (in other words, 75 percent of people with migraine are women). In a simple count, pharmaceutical representations of people with migraine approximate these estimates. However, the placement of representations of the migraine patient on pharmaceutical websites exaggerates this gender disparity. Epidemiological studies also consistently find that migraine is far more prevalent among people with low incomes, yet almost everyone in these advertisements for migraine treatments appears to be middle class or to hold professional positions. Finally, migraine does seem to be a bit more prevalent among whites than blacks, but migraine is not nearly as white a phenomenon as migraine advertisements might lead one to believe. An estimated 9.8 percent of blacks have migraine (versus 12.4 percent of whites) and more blacks than whites (6.1 percent versus 4.25 percent) have what is called "probable migraine"—a diagnosis in which an individual's head pain fits most, but not all, of the guidelines for migraine.[36]

Taken as a whole, these advertisements reinforce a certain image of the typical migraine patient with the general public. If one were to use pharmaceutical advertisements as a guideline for determining who is most likely to get migraine, the conclusion would be a white middle-class woman, attractive, with styled hair, expensive-looking clothing, jewelry, and well-applied makeup. One might also conclude that migraine is not a disabling disease, since in migraine advertisements, anyone with migraine could take a pill and resume going about her day, whether at work, play, or at home. This message underscores a fundamental disparity in the public's understanding of migraine: migraine may be real, but it is certainly not serious. That is, while the existence of a drug like Imitrex may serve to underscore the biological reality of migraine, it has done little to promote migraine as a serious illness. Morever, the marketing of triptans has perpetuated a highly gendered vision of who gets migraine.

Marketing Migraine as a Feminine Experience

Why does the pharmaceutical industry depict migraine as a women's condition when a huge number of men (an estimated 6 percent of the US adult male population) also get migraine? While common sense suggests that the industry is undercutting potential sales of its own drugs, it might be good business practice to stick with the demographic that already seeks help from doctors and which, as many medical sociologists have pointed out, is easier to medicalize and represents the proverbial "low hanging fruit" of consumption.[37] This is a common practice with many drugs, not just those for migraine. However, just because it is common does not mean that it's not problematic.

The marketing principle in action here is called "market segmentation." Because it is both impractical and unwise to design a promotional campaign that appeals to a broad audience, marketers have learned to divide potential customers into sectors thought to hold a coherent set of attitudes, beliefs, or desires. Markets can segment in various ways: *geographic* segmentation divides markets into groups by nations, regions, cities, or states; *psychographic* segmentation divides markets into groups based on values, social class, lifestyle, or personality characteristics; *behavioral* segmentation divides markets based on consumer knowledge or attitudes; while *demographic* segmentation divides markets based on gender, race, family size, income, education, or nationality. The resulting advertisements make it seem natural that the target market should use the advertised product. For example, through market segmentation and gendered advertising, minivans, laundry, and dieting seem to be more feminine, while Jeeps, cigars, and muscles are more masculine. As counterintuitive as it may seem, companies make more money when they divvy up these products and sell them to a smaller audience. One might also argue that migraine drugs are different than minivans, in that there is no equivalent "male" drug to sell to men with migraine, in the way that "Jeeps" offer a male alternative to minivans. But advertisers are bean counters: if they must choose whether to represent the patient as a man or woman, they will choose the representation that will sell the most drugs. Women seek more care and have more migraines, making the choice obvious from a business perspective. Although the gender essentialism perpetuated in migraine advertisements is epiphenomenal to business practices, naturalizing the relationship between migraine and a particular kind of woman exacerbates the legitimacy deficit.

In addition to representing migraine as a women's condition, the pharmaceutical industry engages in a liberal use of gendered metaphors in its effort to connect migraine to women. Metaphors, which connect an abstract idea to something concrete and familiar, are useful when trying to communicate something difficult to represent, as bodily symptoms often are.[38] Advertisements for antihistamines, for example, will show fields of flowers to indicate that the drug will give the consumer a renewed ability to enjoy the natural world. Metaphors can work the other way, too, such that the product can stand in as a concrete representation for something abstract, such as the way that advertisers have linked diamonds to romance and alcohol to the promise of sex. Indeed, when metaphors work well, the product itself becomes a metaphor for these otherwise abstract notions. Marketers use metaphors to draw upon cultural values and tropes to sell their products.

Migraine promotions use gendered metaphors, like the "lost day," to communicate the disability associated with migraine. For example, to promote the use of Botox to treat chronic migraine, Allergan ran a promotion called "Rewrite Your Day," which focused on moments that people with chronic migraine had "lost" to their disease. The centerpiece of this promotion was a contest, in which Allergan asked people living with chronic migraine to submit stories of events missed because of symptoms. Winners received a special event created for them by a celebrity event planner. In itself, the metaphor of a lost day is broadly applicable, but the implementation of this promotion was highly feminized. The website through which contestants were asked to submit their stories, for example, was designed with pink text. Examples of events that could be relived included traditionally feminine fantasies, like weddings and anniversaries. No mention was made of significant lost days that might appeal to men, for example, a missed hunting trip, football game, or corporate event—or even just a day earning much-needed wages. The first winner, a woman named Patrice Johnson, described her wedding day in her story: "I spent months perfecting every detail—from the original centerpieces to the homemade food—so not being able to enjoy my wedding day was beyond disappointing. I even wrote personal vows, but I rushed through them at the altar since the migraine made it uncomfortable to read."[39] Allergan's promotion turns on a Cinderella fantasy in which a fairy godmother grants fairy tale moments to people with chronic migraine.

Pfizer drew upon a similarly feminized metaphor in a 2003 campaign that compared the act of taking its migraine drug, Relpax (eletriptan), to a spa experience. According to coverage in *Medical Marketing and Media*, as part of this marketing strategy, "Pfizer turned a wing of New York's Grand Central Terminal into a 'soothing oasis dedicated to the five senses' in a consumer promotion last month for its migraine headache medication Relpax":[40] "The one-day event, which began at 7 a.m. and continued until 8 p.m., attracted thousands of commuters. The spa area included a three-piece orchestra, yoga clinics, a free massage area, a Zen garden, and a gourmet food sampling area. Interspersed among these areas were Internet kiosks and Relpax posters with slogans such as 'Thanks to Relpax I'm ready to step out again.' . . . Consumers who filled out a short survey about migraines received a gift carton that included a Relpax pamphlet, tea sample, scented candle and a mini eyelid mask."[41] Consumers were sent to kiosks where they could access the Relpax website, which featured a "virtual spa." This spa, a small pop-up window, played soothing sounds of a rain forest accompanied by images evocative of a spa vacation. Across the screen, the text used "spa experience" as a metaphor to describe the pain of migraine. For example, the text read:

> **Imagine the fresh scent of a beautiful garden.** For some, even the most exhilarating fragrance can increase nausea when the pain of a full-blown migraine takes over.
>
> **Imagine the gentle touch of your dancing partner.** Even a soft touch that causes the slightest motion can become unbearable. Sometimes, that's how it feels when you're stopped in your tracks by headsplitting migraine pain.[42]

Both of these promotions pitch migraine drugs as lifestyle drugs, when, in fact, migraine devastates lives. While Allergan's "lost day" promotion emphasizes the disability associated with migraine, it also presumes that a person with chronic migraine could reschedule and relive this missed event. But the problem with chronic migraine is that it persists, making it difficult for people who have it to make and keep plans. Likewise, luxury spas, with their migraine-triggering scents, are a difficult place for many people with episodic or chronic migraine. Indeed, the Relpax promotion distributed several migraine triggers in the service of advertising their drug. Many people with migraine cannot drink tea, avoid many kinds of food, and dread the perfume of scented candles. Even the metaphor about gardens gets the experience of migraine wrong. While it's true that a migraine attack can heighten one's sensitivity to certain smells (as in the example of an "exhilarating fragrance" that "can increase nausea when the pain of a full-blown migraine takes over"), fragrances are often a migraine trigger, meaning they trigger migraine in the first place. I believe that I speak for many people with migraine when I say that an "exhilarating fragrance" is often both nauseating and painful at any time, whether one has a migraine or not.

Both the "Rewrite Your Day" contest and the spa metaphor draw upon feminized cultural tropes to reinforce ubiquitous images of middle-class women as archetypal migraine patients. They represent the migraine experience as essentially feminine, when, indeed, nothing inherent to the experience of migraine is feminine. Moreover, the promotions present migraine as a problem of the leisure class—a problem for people for whom it might be relevant to be offered contest prizes like "event planning" and gifts like eyelid masks.

Migraines as a Flaw of Moral Character

Advertising strategies also rely on a standard narrative that positions migraine as an obstacle to women's ability to nurture and care. In these narratives, women in the throes of a migraine attack are portrayed as uncaring, difficult, and agitated, bordering on hysterical. Migraine medications are then presented as not just a treatment for the symptoms of migraine, but as a solution to the moral dilemmas posed by migraine. In this last section of the chapter, I describe three such campaigns, organized by two different companies, GSK and AstraZeneca.

The first campaign, run by GSK to promote Imitrex, features a small booklet that includes information on the drug—for example, it explains how Imitrex differs from general analgesics and describes how one should ask a physician for the medication. Alongside this information, the booklet tells a visual story of a young white woman's recovery from a migraine. This story, it should be noted, has almost no connection with the information provided about Imitrex in the pages interspersed between these images. It begins with the woman standing confidently next to a floating

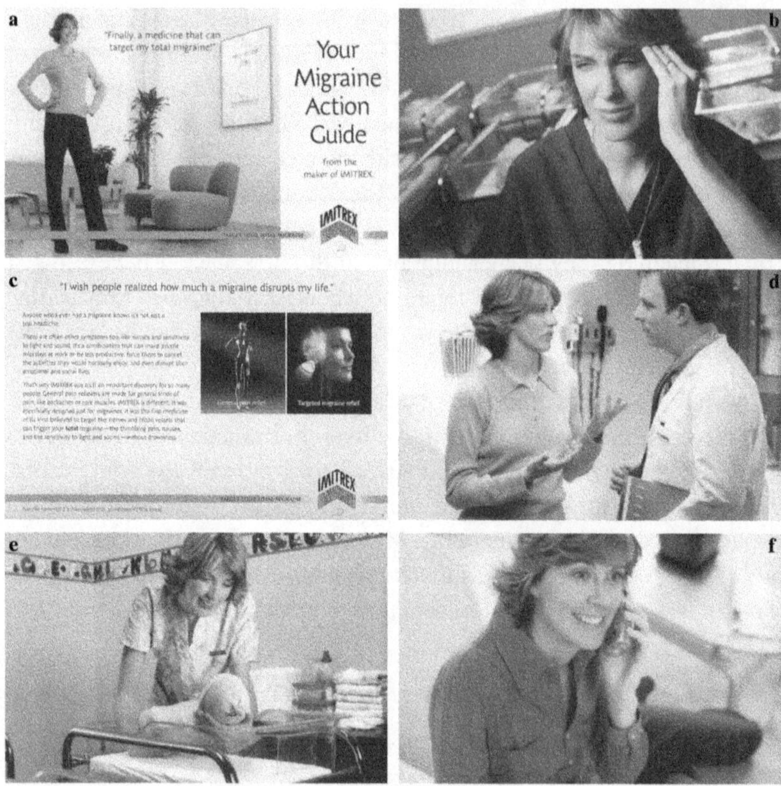

FIGURE 4.1 a–f: Imitrex advertisement.

quotation that narrates her thoughts, "Finally, a medicine that can target my total migraine!" (see figure 4.1a). On the inside cover, she reappears, this time dressed in a nurse's uniform, working in a hospital room full of newborn infants. But she is in pain. She grimaces, presses her fingers into her temple, and furrows her brow. Her back is turned away from the babies, presumably because the intensity of the pain disables her and prevents her from performing her job. Because her job is in a neonatal ward, this means that she is neglecting rows and rows of babies. That the marketers chose to represent their model migraine patient as a neonatal nurse manages to elicit feminine qualities of nurture and care, while resonating with mothers' guilt for failing to care for children when they, too, feel ill.

The nurse gives voice to her frustration on the top of the next page: "I wish people realized how much a migraine disrupts my life" (see figure 4.1c). Imitrex is proposed as the proper solution. The text explains: "General pain relievers are made for general kinds of pain . . . IMITREX is different." Using a computer-animated outline of a universal patient (enlarged in figure 4.1c), the image depicts how Imitrex works. The universal patient used here is a woman, rather than the typical "universal man" so often used to portray the medical norm.[43] The spots on the first body demonstrate how diffuse general pain relief can be. The adjacent image demonstrates how Imitrex works differently, by "targeting" the pain. Here, we see one of the few images in any advertisement that alludes to a biological basis for migraine. Shaped like a bullet, the tablet shoots toward the source of the pain, targeting only the brain. Not surprisingly, specificity is a trait that people value in their drugs.[44] Specificity is also the trait that has led headache specialists to credit Imitrex with legitimating migraine as a real, biological condition.

The nurse is delighted that Imitrex can help. Armed with this new knowledge, she approaches her physician for a prescription (see figure 4.1d). She gesticulates animatedly, and the physician (a white male) appears to listen actively, his posture signifying relinquished authority and an attentive respect for the patient's medical insight. The two are positioned at nearly the same height, signaling shared power in the interaction. The advertisement seeks to empower patients to bring this new information straight to their physician.

The physician must have prescribed Imitrex because in the next two images (figures 4.1e and 4.1f), she is free of pain and back to work. With Imitrex, the neonatal ward no longer carries the cold, institutionalized ambience of the earlier picture and now looks more like a homey nursery. Warm, yellow walls with alphabet bordering signal a change in atmosphere. The nurse's demeanor has changed as well. She now cradles and cares for a baby, tenderly smiling and cooing. She has a renewed capacity for care work. Not only has she returned to her work of nurturing babies, she has returned to her social life, and is presumably telling her friends how terrific Imitrex is. In short, the patient is a happy customer, restored to life by GSK's medication.

This visual narrative appeals to the consumer by using images that draw on culturally resonant images of women at work. Stories have more rhetorical force when they are relevant to beliefs already held by the audience.[45] Advertisements that coincide with broadly held commonsense notions about the ways of the world appear to be natural and objective. By setting this narrative in a neonatal ward, the advertisement is designed to appeal to women at work and at home with their children. The manifest message of these images is that the medication is effective and that those with migraine should communicate this information to their physicians at their next consultation. The latent message, on the other hand, confirms that migraine is a women's disorder that disrupts feminine efforts to care for others. Imitrex transforms this woman from a person who cannot cope with her everyday life to a warm, engaging, friendly presence. The pill does more than treat her migraine symptoms; it transforms her into a more reasonable, dependable person.

Guilt is an effective and pervasive tool used throughout migraine advertisements. It's a gendered form of guilt: like the nurse who cannot care for babies when she is in pain, or women in the throes of migraine who are depicted as bad mothers because they are prevented from giving their children the care they need. Disabled by their migraine, they appear to abandon their children, literally turning their back on their kids. For example, in a Zomig (zolmitriptan) advertisement that effectively exploits this narrative, a woman sits in pain on a bus (see figure 4.2). She is experiencing stress—both the daily stress of motherhood and the stress of running errands while caring for her son. Like the mother in the previous advertisement, her body posture is turned away from her child. Her right hand pressing against her temple may soothe the pain, but it also shields him from her sight. Her opposite hand reaches around her body to hold on to his arm, perhaps signaling a residual desire to nurture. Yet the headline "Escape" evokes a more primal desire of liberation from an overwhelming day-to-day routine. One gets the sense that motherhood might be too much to bear. Zomig is positioned as the treatment, not just for migraine symptoms, but for life. Zomig allows women to return to their maternal duties.

These advertisements depend on a narrative of transformation in which a person becomes whole through medication. The woman transformed by migraine medication is what anthropologist Emily Martin might describe as a "pharmaceutical person," or someone whose personality is mediated and, in some ways, completed, via the drugs that she takes.[46] Martin describes this transformation vis-à-vis psychopharmaceuticals, in which drugs transform individuals from irrational to rational actors. Even as headache medicine has moved away from a model in which migraine is understood to be a condition of irrationality, this narrative persists in migraine advertisements. Much like Valium in the 1960s, these ads posi-

Escape
from the confines of
migraine pain...
www.ZOMIG.com

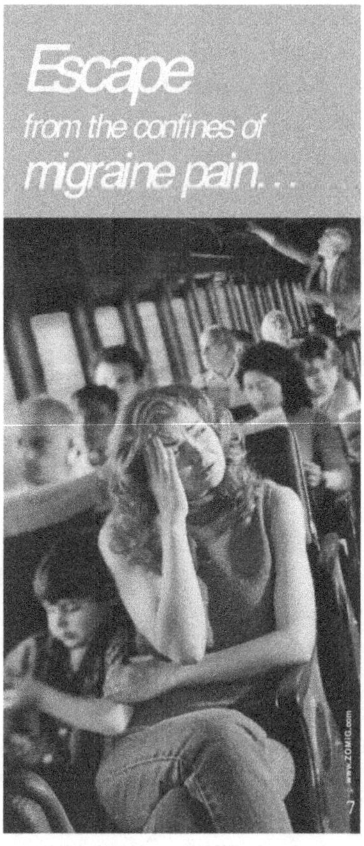

FIGURE 4.2 Zomig advertisement "Escape from Migraine." *M, the Magazine for Migraine Management.*

tion Imitrex and Zomig as a version of "mother's little helpers," enabling women to get on with their duties as caregivers.[47]

I saw one particularly striking example of this narrative at work at an elaborate booth set up by AstraZeneca at the 2003 International Headache Congress (IHC) in Rome. At this lavish booth, conference goers (mainly medical professionals who treat migraine patients) were invited to watch the "Migraine Experience." Located just inside the entrance of the grand convention center, AstraZeneca was able to advertise its triptan, Zomig, to the thousands of medical doctors, physician assistants, and psychologists who were in attendance. It was a popular stop along the corridor outside the large auditorium where presenters gave their talks. Other pharmaceutical booths competed for attention by distributing flash drives, mugs, and posters, but the theater, which promised viewers that they could experience a migraine just as their patients might, consistently attracted small groups of attendees.

I joined a small line of about five or six people and wondered as I waited how a virtual migraine would compare to the real experience. After a few moments, an usher led us into a small, dark theater. The room lacked seating, but contained three large screens—one directly to the front, and one to each side—and a red button, which the usher instructed us to press if "there are any problems." The usher closed the door, leaving us in a dark room. There was nothing but silence for a long minute and then a thunderstorm approached in the dark. I wondered whether the storm signified the "nerve storm" thought to occur in the brain during migraine, the fact that weather fronts often trigger migraine, or the mood one might feel during a migraine. Suddenly, the screen lit up, revealing a sunny living room. We saw a brunette woman talking on the phone, while her blond son was playing a game on the sofa. Their television was on and there was a high-pitched, pulsing noise on the soundtrack, suggesting an anxious mood. The woman shouted at her son, "Into the bathroom now! And, don't forget your green swimming trunks!" She then picked up with her phone conversation and said, "My darling husband, hello?"

We heard her husband's voice as he replied cheerily, telling her that all was well on his trip to Venice. He asked after their son, Jack. In contrast to his cheer, she sounded annoyed. "Everything is a competition," she said, and then paused, while she yelled at her son to get ready. Her husband calmly told her to keep her voice down, and she responded with a sigh . . .

"Are you alright? You seem pretty tense. You don't want to get sick again."

"There's no way that I can afford to have a migraine right now. I just haven't got the time. We're really stretched at work. Everyone is really being pushed to their limits."

He made some suggestions, which she dismissed and they hung up. The soundtrack turned ominous again. She looked into a mirror and stared into a distorted reflection of herself. Her forehead pulsed with what seemed to be tension. She walked into the kitchen, where her son sat dressed at the kitchen table. She approached him and softly said, "Jack. Jack . . . I'm really sorry that I shouted at you earlier. I'll fix you a drink and then we'll go, okay?"

Very sweetly, Jack asked to go to the beach. Looking guilty, the mother said she would be too busy with work and added with a trembling voice, "And I'm not feeling . . . too well. Maybe we can go on Friday when Daddy gets home? That would be good, wouldn't it?" As she turned to hand her son his drink, she couldn't quite make it to the table. She put the drink down on the counter, and we saw her son, Jack, from her perspective. Her vision was beginning to fragment, and he was getting blurry. The music was high pitched and eerie. Stumbling now, she said, "Jack? Jack? I don't think I can take you. I can't . . . see . . . to drive. Listen to me. . . . I'll ring grandmom and tell her to come collect you. All right? I just got to lie down for a little while. So, why don't you go to your room and play on your computer. I will call grandmom and she will come. All right?"

In a montage, we saw her lying in bed. Distorted voices swirled over her. We heard her whispering, "No . . . no . . ." We heard an echo of her mother's voice saying that she didn't mind helping. We heard her calling out of work. And, repeatedly we heard her son's voice, saying, "Mommy" and the image of him bringing her a drink. But the scene was blurry and confused, depicting a phantasmagoric sequence of images and sound. We saw and heard her vomit. As the music became calmer, she emerged from her room and down the stairs. She was disheveled, wearing only a long T-shirt. Her hair was loose around her face, and she dripped with sweat. She was worried.

"Jack?" She called out for her son, "Jack?" Increasingly frantic, she called out, "Jack! Answer me! Where are you? Jack!" Just then, the phone rang. She picked up and heard her mother. She said, "Mum, I can't find Jack. I don't know where he is." The music became calmer, as the grandmother told her that she had Jack. "You rang me, don't you remember?" She put Jack on the phone, and he asked his mother if she was okay.

She assured her son that she was okay and asked about his day. He was fine, and she promised to take him to the beach on the weekend. He replied, "You won't get sick again . . ."

"No, no darling. I won't get sick."

"Promise mommy!"

The music lightened and the screen switched to Zomig's logo.

The whole film takes just a few minutes, but the message is clear. The woman, disorientated and distressed by her migraine symptoms, cannot properly care for her son. When she emerges from her room a few hours later, she endures every mother's worst nightmare: the fear that she has lost her child. Though on this occasion she managed to call her mother for help, the film suggests that she might not be so lucky next time. The mother also misses valuable work time because of her migraine, but this loss is only touched on briefly in the story. By far the greatest emphasis is on her failed duties as a mother. Like the print advertisements, the narrative leads viewers to believe that her lapse in care is not a one-off occurrence, but a recurring and destructive part of her ordinary life. We are keyed into her personality when she moves in an instant from saccharine "My darling husband, hello!" to difficult "Everything is a challenge." Her husband, a calm—if distant—presence in the house, senses immediately that she is overwhelmed and requests that she relax and ask for help, lest she "get sick again." But the woman refuses to listen to his advice and is almost immediately struck down with a migraine—a migraine very clearly caused by the overwhelming stress in her life. Her migraine disrupts the family and very nearly causes the woman to put their child in danger. This is a narrative reminiscent of antidepressant advertisements from the 1960s, which presented women as uncontrollable threats to their husband and children.[48] And like more recent advertisements for Prozac, AstraZeneca's migraine medication offers a remedy to placate the woman and improve her efficiency as a homemaker.

The film derives its power from its ability to reflect and construct a particular reality, in which women's primary duty is to care for children—a duty assumed to be straightforward for pain-free women. Men are not represented as caretakers, nor are they represented as sufferers of migraine. This kind of marketing material provides a detailed and emotive social context in which women have migraine, and in which their symptoms have damaging effects on their loved ones. No similar context is imagined for men.

Guilt, one pharmaceutical executive explained to me, is a common theme that emerges in industry-sponsored focus groups of women with migraine. Women with migraine report that they feel inadequate as mothers, as wives, and as employees when they have attacks. From the executive's perspective, she and other pharmaceutical companies were providing a service: a way to enable women to perform their duties. But their advertising is darker than that. By playing on these very fears to create their market, pharmaceutical advertisements create normative expectations for how women in pain behave and how quickly they ought to recover.

Take an Imitrex and Call Me in the Morning

The pharmaceutical industry and its products have played a central role in bettering the lives of millions of people with migraine. New migraine drugs helped foster the paradigmatic shift that transformed migraine from a psychosomatic condition of the mind to a neurobiological disease of the brain. For migraine researchers, the pharmaceutical industry has been a savior, supplying their community with hundreds of millions of dollars in research and educational funds. For men and women with migraine, myself included, triptans delivered much-needed relief, all while providing "proof" that our migraines were real. And yet, it is important to remember that, in exchange for these goods, the industry has received an immense amount of power to determine what we know about and how we understand migraine. For all the good that the pharmaceutical industry has done, its values are tied up with the values of generating economic wealth.

The vision of migraine perpetuated by the pharmaceutical industry might be good for selling drugs, but it also perpetuates the legitimacy deficit. The focus on portraying migraine as a white woman's problem reflects, in part, both an epidemiological and clinical reality: more women than men get migraine and more women than men seek help for head pain. But these advertisements render invisible everyone else who has migraine. Six percent of the US adult male population has migraine. More men experience migraine than diseases of the prostate and ulcers combined, all of which are described and constructed as either specifically male diseases or unisex.[49] Marketers may want to target women because women buy more of their medication; but by using gendered frameworks like carework, guilt, and princess moments, drug companies may actually perpetuate the stereotypes that keep people from taking migraine seriously.

Not surprisingly, the depiction of migraine propagated in pharmaceutical marketing materials has little to nothing to say about socioeconomic status. The fantasy embedded in migraine advertisements is that the suffering wrought by migraine is temporary and distinctly bourgeois. Relief is a commodity bought and sold at the local pharmacy. But this restitution narrative is too easy. For one thing, these drugs are not as readily available as depicted. As prescription drugs, migraine medications depend on access to physicians who understand migraine and who are willing to treat it. And the cost of migraine drugs remains prohibitive. Before going off patent, Imitrex cost $27 per pill, and it took one to two pills per migraine attack to treat it.[50] The price of Imitrex has dropped considerably since its patent expired, but GSK is now promoting in its place a new drug called Treximet, which still costs about $20 per pill. Treximet is a combination of sumatriptan (the active drug in Imitrex) and naproxen (a nonsteroidal anti-inflammatory drug that is available over the counter under the brand name of Aleve). Botox, the latest drug to be approved by the FDA for the treatment of chronic migraine, costs $600–$1,000 and is administered every three months. These drugs are not practically available to those without access to physicians and prescription drug insurance plans.

But restitution would remain elusive, even if these drugs were free. The truth is that, over the last forty years, *only one class of medications*—triptans—has been developed specifically to treat migraines. And triptans, while very effective for some people, are only moderately more effective than Excedrin, the over-the-counter mix of aspirin, acetaminophen, and caffeine that has long been available. The very best drugs available for the prevention of migraine—like Topamax—only reduce the incidence of migraine by 50 percent in 50 percent of the people who take them. The pharmaceutical industry has a long way to go before migraine is "easy to treat."

The restitution narrative creates problems for all people with migraine, no matter what their race, class, or gender. By suggesting that migraine is so easy to treat, these advertisements omit the millions of people for whom these drugs are not effective or, worse, for whom these drugs have iatrogenic effects. Physicians now say that any abortive drug taken more than twice per week can cause "medication overuse headache," in which migraine transforms into a more chronic form of head pain. Withdrawing the offending medication can usually treat this iatrogenic condition, but in some cases, the now-daily migraine will not relent. But one would never know from advertisements that the very drug for sale can cause even more pain or that, drug or no drug, migraine can be a horrifying, disabling condition for which treatment is difficult to obtain. Instead, drug advertisements are cavalier, offering a modern-day translation of the kind of advice doctors give when they aren't too concerned: "Take an Imitrex and call me in the morning."

Imagine living with an intractable form of chronic migraine in a world in which these advertisements dominate public consciousness. When health fails to improve despite the availability of "revolutionary" drugs like Imitrex, patients may experience a form of double jeopardy—not only do they live with untreatable chronic pain, but their inability to get better might be read as a failure of moral character. In other words, if headache drugs are represented as a salve, capable of restoring a patient to a "whole woman," then what happens to the patient who doesn't respond to drugs, as is the case with a large proportion of people with migraine?[51]

All people with migraine—men and women—are diminished because the portrayal of women in migraine advertisements elicits historical associations between pain, hysteria, and neurotic women. By using metaphors, imagery, and narratives that exploit and reify gender stereotypes about motherhood and guilt, pain and weakness, stress and coping, migraine advertisements risk stigmatizing both men and women who have migraine. Although the pharmaceutical industry has produced good products that help millions of people, the marriage of pharmaceutical industry, advertising, and profits has unwittingly led to the diminution of migraine as a disease.

CHAPTER FIVE

Men in Pain

In her classic essay, "If Men Could Menstruate," Gloria Steinem proposes that, in such a world, men would brag about how much they bleed and how long the bleeding lasts, the government would organize a National Institute of Dysmenorrhea, and menstrual pads and tampons would be federally funded and free: "Statistical surveys would show that men did better in sports and won more Olympic medals during their periods. Generals, right-wing politicians, and religious fundamentalists would cite menstruation ('*men*-struation') as proof that only men could serve God and country in combat ('You have to give blood to take blood'), occupy high political office ('Can women be properly fierce without a monthly cycle governed by the planet Mars?'), be priests, ministers, God Himself ('He gave this blood for our sins'), or rabbis ('Without a monthly purge of impurities, women are unclean')." In short, "whatever a 'superior' group has will be used to justify its superiority, and whatever an 'inferior' group has will be used to justify its plight."[1]

Steinem's tongue-in-cheek poke at role reversal raises fundamental questions about headache disorders. Migraine is generally understood as a women's disease despite the fact that men also get migraine. In this book, I have argued that this gendering is pervasive, persistently embedded in neurobiological models of migraine and reproduced in pharmaceutical representations of the disorder. On the other hand, one might argue that the feminization of migraine is merely reflective of an objective reality in which "migraine brains" truly are "sensitive." In this chapter, I imagine how migraines might be understood if they were assumed to be a men's disease. Would medical descriptions of the disorder look different? Would patients experience more social or medical legitimation?

Cluster headache offers a glimpse of what such a world might look like.

Like migraine, cluster headache is a pain disorder that causes tremendous disability. Both disorders are accompanied by severe head pain, and both disorders are treated with a similar (although not an identical) pharmacopeia. Unlike migraine, cluster headache affects more men than women. Epidemiological research on the condition is sparse and ever changing, but current estimates suggest that men experience cluster headache between two to three times more often than women.[2]

While both headache disorders cause pain, they are not the same. Cluster headache is an unusually dramatic disorder. Its signature symptom is a one-sided, severe headache, which many call the worst pain one can experience.[3] The pain itself is located around the eye and burns with a quality that people with cluster headache compare to "a hot poker in the eye,"[4] or more vividly to a "metal spike being pounded into [the] eye and pushed through the skull, deep into [the] brain."[5] The pain is often accompanied by a variety of autonomic nervous symptoms: red, swollen, droopy, and tearing eyes; a congested or runny nose; forehead and facial sweating; pupil dilation or contraction.[6] In addition, cluster headaches provoke restless behavior. In the midst of an attack, people with cluster headache will pace, jump, or even bang their heads against the wall to find relief. Whereas migraine is very common, cluster headache is relatively rare, affecting less than 1 percent of the population.[7] Many people with cluster headache have never met anyone else with the same disorder. However, although migraine and cluster headache are different disorders, there is clearly overlap between these diagnoses. For example, women with cluster headache tend to have migrainous symptoms with their attacks, including nausea and light sensitivity.

What makes cluster headache so provocative is the extent to which its epidemiology is encoded in medical descriptions of the disorder. Unlike migraine, metaphors of masculinity—not femininity—guide scientific and nonscientific understandings of cluster headache. Take, for example, this fairly typical medical description of cluster headache, written by three leading headache specialists: "Cluster headache is probably the most dramatic of all the headache types. . . . Cluster pain is so excruciating that it brings even the strongest of men to their knees. . . . Rather than retreating to a dark, quiet room, as do migraine sufferers, cluster patients cannot sit or lie still. Rather, they pace, rock, and drive their fists into the painful eye. Some patients may even show unusual behavior, such as hitting themselves in the head, banging their heads against the wall, or engaging in intense physical activity such as push-ups or running."[8] The gender ideology embedded within this description is explicit. The authors use everyday notions of masculinity to convey the epidemiological "fact" that cluster headache tends to affect men. Their choice to use the image of "the strongest of men" on their knees reinforces the intensity of cluster pain and its predominance among men, while making clear that there is nothing weak or feminine about having the disorder. The fundamental masculinity of cluster headache is further invoked by comparing its aggressive symptoms to the passive retreat of migraine—cluster headache does not share the femininity of its diagnostic cousin.

I have traced this masculinized language back to the late 1960s, when physicians began describing cluster headache not just as a disorder predominant in men, but as a disorder of *excess* masculinity. Since then, stereotypical cluster patients have been described as "hyper-masculine,"[9] "mesomorphs" with lion-like facial features[10] who are "masculinized in behavior and habit."[11] This masculine discourse even extends to female cluster headache patients, who are recast as women who lack feminine qualities or whose bodies are punishing them for transgressing traditional gender roles.[12] This physical and psychological description of cluster headache ("the cluster profile") has been remarkably resilient over time, even though more recent studies do not support this profile.

The exaggerated masculinization in descriptions of cluster headache—its predominance among men, its dramatic and sometimes violent symptomatic expression, and its folkloric status as a disorder of the hyper-masculine—provides a rich contrast to migraine and an intriguing comparative case for understanding how the gendering of disorders occurs and how this gendering shapes the collective recognition of specific diseases as serious, real, and worthy of social investment. Cluster headache serves as an "extreme" case of medicalized masculinity, magnifying the processes of gendering and bringing into relief features of the world whose routine operation we might otherwise overlook.[13] Examining the masculinity in cluster headache demonstrates the contingency of the language and metaphors we use to understand and construct biological processes underlying pain, particularly as similar phenomena in migraine and cluster headache are described so differently. Finally, the persistence of masculinity embedded in the cluster headache literature in a time of increasing gender sensitivity elsewhere in medicine demands an explanation. Explaining why researchers and advocates view the masculinity of cluster headache as unproblematic reveals the immense value ascribed to these moral characteristics. Medicalized masculinity is embraced, I argue, because it confers status on both physicians and patients. Nevertheless, this masculinity is not sufficient to fully close cluster headache's legitimacy deficit. As I discuss later in the chapter, people with cluster headache still struggle to convince others that their disorder is different from headache or migraine, which they see as feminine styles of pain that are easier to control.

This case study begins by highlighting the masculinity embedded in symptomatic accounts of cluster headache. I then move toward a historical analysis to examine how cluster headache, as a diagnosis, transformed from a condition that disproportionately affects men to a condition conceived as a disorder of masculinity. I ask, to what extent does this profile still exist? What explains the persistent presence of masculinity in the models these researchers deploy? Most importantly, what can cluster headache teach us about the relationship between gender and legitimacy in illness?

Gendering the Language of Cluster Pain

By all accounts, cluster headache is extraordinarily painful. Patients describe the quality of the pain as boring, piercing, or burning, as opposed to the throbbing pain of migraine. Joel Saper and Kenneth Magee relay these descriptions from their patients: "[One patient said it felt] as though the skin of his face and his eyes were being clawed from his skull and acid poured into the open wound. Another victim described the attacks as a burning metal spike being pounded into his eye and pushed through the skull, deep into his brain. One patient likened his attacks to the flame of a blowtorch being applied to his eye for fifteen to twenty minutes."[14] Lee Kudrow, a headache specialist who has cluster headaches, described his own pain as "a 'force' pushing with such incredible power through my eye that my head appears to be moving backward, yielding to its resistance."[15] Bill Pahlow of the now-defunct Organization for Understanding Cluster Headache (OUCH) told me that cluster headache "literally feels like somebody stuck a red hot screwdriver in your eyeball . . . and just twists it around." DJ, another cluster headache advocate, describes the pain as the worst he ever had: "Literally, [it's] like someone drives a railroad spike in your eye and while it's in there just kind of shoves it around or kind of twists it around, whatever you want to say. . . . I've had two brain surgeries now for a different condition that I would have any day versus having another cluster headache."

The extraordinary nature of cluster headaches is highlighted by the behavior associated with the disorder. People with cluster headache are restless and sometimes violent toward themselves during attacks. The restlessness of those with cluster headache is widely recognized; some neurologists suggest that "agitation, restlessness, or absence of aggravation of pain with movement" be added to the IHS diagnostic criteria as an additional differential feature.[16] This is a far cry from the "sensitive" migraine patient, who escapes her pain through retreat—hiding in a dark, quiet room. Headache specialists, at present, believe that these highly gendered reactions are not determined by gender at all, but are universal features generated by internal biological mechanisms. For cluster headache, the most likely candidate is the hypothalamus, a part of the brain that responds to movement.

Biological theories, aside, the particular language used to describe the movement made by those with cluster headache is rooted within cultural norms of masculinity. Banging heads and fists are only partly biologically determined behaviors; in large part, such behavior is strongly shaped by cultural expectations of what it means to be male. There may be good biological reasons why movement alleviates the pain of cluster headache, but the specific forms that this movement takes might also be culturally determined. The fact that the aggression of cluster headache (e.g., punching one's head) fits with typically masculine behavior contributes to a vision of cluster headache as a prototypically male disorder.

This masculinity is exacerbated when descriptions of this aggressive behavior are suffused with normative bravado, as if the violence of the pain must be matched by equally violent behavior. Consider, for example, the following excerpt from a patient narrative posted to clusterheadaches.com:

> It's somewhere between 11:00 P.M. and 3:00 A.M., and I wake terrified, hopeful that I'm dreaming, and knowing that I'm not. I move quickly out of bed while my lovely wife of fifteen years, the only one who truly tries to understand, watches helpless; as there is nothing that she can do, she hurts too. I am careful not to wake the children as I make my way down the stairs. If they were to witness my nightly cluster ritual, they would never see me the same way again. Their father, fearless protector, diligent provider, crawling about in tears, beating his head on the hard wood floor.
>
> The pain is so intense I want to scream, but I never do. I go down three flights of stairs where I can't be heard, and drop to my knees. I place my hands

> on the back of my neck, and lock my fingers together. I bind my head between my arms and squeeze as hard as I can in an attempt to crush my scull. . . . I search for the telephone that has always been my weapon of choice for creating a diversion, and I beat my left temple with the hand piece. I create a rhythm as I strike my scull, cursing the demon with each blow. I reach a point of distraction from the cluster, and then I start the whole process over; roll and squeeze, crawl and bang, find the telephone.[17]

This person, obviously in tremendous pain, describes his experiences from a distinctly masculine perspective. He is married with children, and worries that he will lose their respect as their "fearless protector" and "diligent provider." But the masculinity in this narrative is not limited to his social role. Rather, it dominates his whole experience of the pain. For example, the author attempts to "crush" his pain by way of his own strength. He describes his desperate search for the telephone, which he uses to beat the "demon." The telephone is his "weapon of choice."

The Internet community on clusterheadaches.com terms this restless behavior "the dance," an ironic reference to "headbanging." More subtly, the dance also references the quick steps a boxer takes as he circles his opponent, which in this case is often referred to as the "demon" or the "beast." Imagining the pain as a combatant is common in cluster headache narratives, in dramatic contrast to the metaphors of waiting, hiding, and retreating so often seen in migraine narratives.

Occasionally, participants in cluster headache newsgroups ask each other whether anything hurts worse than a cluster headache. Men write in war stories of shattered bones and gangrene limbs that pale in comparison to a cluster attack. Headache specialist Peter Goadsby writes that of the cluster headache patients in his clinic, "none has recalled a worse pain than headache."[18] Indeed, more than one male physician told me that women with cluster headache describe the pain as "worse than childbirth." Pahlow confirmed that "the ladies [in OUCH] that have it say it's worse than giving birth." These comparisons capitalize on the cultural currency of childbirth, using it as a gold standard of pain, immediately recognizable by all as an excruciating experience.[19] Those who experience cluster headaches have adopted the nickname "suicide headache" to highlight the violence embedded within the cluster experience. Many people with cluster headache either contemplate suicide in fear of another attack or beg to be killed during an attack. Some people with cluster headache do commit suicide (as do some people with migraine), and clinic-based studies have found that suicidal ideation is more frequent among cluster headache patients during an attack than it is for other headache patients.[20]

There is no doubt that cluster headache is a real, immediate, and traumatizing pain disorder. What is curious is the way it has been spun into a disorder of masculinity within the medical literature. The next section describes the historical process through which this has happened. Highlighting the process through which masculinity has been medicalized in cluster headache medicine points to the ways in which masculine descriptions of cluster headache are not inevitable and natural, but rather constructed and negotiated.

From a Men's Disorder to a Disorder of Excess Masculinity

Compared to migraine, cluster headache is a relatively new diagnostic category, emerging in the medical literature in the early twentieth century. Bayard T. Horton and his colleagues at the Mayo Clinic are credited with popularizing the diagnosis of cluster headache in a 1939 article, calling it "erythomelalgia," before switching in 1941 to a new name, "histaminic cephalalgia." But several neurologists with an interest in history have claimed that descriptions of cluster-like pain extend as far back as the clinical notes written by Nicolaes Tulp in 1641.[21] Another early account appears in Gerhard van Swieten's medical textbook written in 1745.[22] Other neurologists suggest cluster headache existed in the literature for centuries, but appeared under a number of alternate names, including histamine headache, Horton's headache, cephalalgia, ciliary neuralgia, cluster-migraine, spenopalatine neuralgia, erythromelalgia, and histamine cephalalgia.[23]

In 1954, E. Charles Kunkle coined the term "cluster headache" to describe the peculiar circadian and circannual rhythm of the disorder.[24] Those with episodic cluster headache have attacks in "cluster periods" or "bouts" that last several weeks or months and which recur seasonally. In addition, individual attacks often have a rhythm, typically occurring at the same time each day. Patients report weeks of daily cluster attacks at 3:00 a.m. so regularly that some refer to the condition as "alarm clock headaches." (A term that conveys that the cycle is rational—a rationality that is absent in discussions of menstrual migraine, which also have cyclic and predictable onset.)[25]

Over time, physicians developed a "cluster profile" that described both the physical and psychological characteristics purportedly associated with this diagnosis. The development of this profile owes a great deal to historical accident, since Horton's introduction of cluster headache coincided with the rise of the psychosomatic movement in medicine. (The first issue of *Psychosomatic Medicine* was also published in 1939.) At about the same time as Horton's discovery, Harold G. Wolff was beginning to develop his own theory of the migraine personality, in which he argued that people with migraine were tense, anxious, and hardworking to a fault (see chapter 1).

Wolff generally thought of cluster headache as a variant of migraine and, thus, considered people with cluster headache to be subject to all of the same personality traits as those with migraine: that is, ambitious, successful, perfectionist, and efficient. Nevertheless, Wolff anticipated the development of a specific cluster headache personality, even providing what might be called the first description of a cluster psyche. Generalizing from one case study, Wolff describes a cluster patient who "was found to be a tense, anxious, extremely conscientious, meticulous, shy, ingoing person with perfectionist and 'just-so' attitudes. He was easily made to feel guilty. He called himself a 'rugged individualist' who literally got a 'headache' when he thought about the 'political situation.' He felt dissatisfied with his work life. He became tense in the presence of most people and was bored by most of his social obligations."[26] Wolff's description varied little from his theories about a migraine personality, but he thought it was important to distinguish between the two. Wolff warned his colleagues to pay close attention to the life situation of their cluster patients, as he believed that strong emotional events could trigger a series of cluster headache attacks.

Arthur Friedman, drawing on then-popular psychoanalytic and personality-based theories, described the typical cluster headache patient as "an adult who was ambitious, efficient, and over-conscientious, strove for perfection, and had a strong tendency toward compulsive behavior. . . . They often had positions of responsibility but were insecure and often had a lack of self-confidence in their ability. The most frequent conflicts observed were of a hostile and aggressive nature."[27] At first glance, Friedman's cluster headache personality is similar to Wolff's migraine personality. Like Wolff's migraine personality, the cluster personality could apply to many kinds of people and lacked useful specificity. And like the migraine personality, the cluster personality medicalized masculine characteristics like ambition, perfectionism, and efficiency—an impression that probably came from the same clinical bias that led to Wolff's initial formulation of the migraine personality. Only the wealthiest and most educated patients would be able to see Friedman in his New York clinic at Montefiore, which may be why he reported that cluster headache patients had all held executive or professional-level occupations. But one psychological feature distinguished the cluster patient from migraine patients. Where Wolff described people with migraine as assertive and productive, Friedman described his cluster patients as aggressive and hostile. The aggression developed, Friedman argued, from a conflict arising between a strong (and masculine) exterior and an insecure, weak interior.

But, in the coming years, Friedman's ideas about the cluster personality found little empirical support. Although a few 1960s-era studies looked for psychological contributions to cluster headache, none had observed unusual levels of abnormal psychological disorders in their patients.[28] Indeed, Friedman's cluster headache profile faced skepticism until 1969, when John R. Graham, another of Wolff's students, presented his research on the cluster personality at a symposium.[29]

Graham embraced Wolff's psychosomatic approach to understanding headache disorders. He described the cluster headache patient as a person with masculine tendencies: "ambitious, hard-working, and [with] a strong sense of social mobility. They push until they break with symptoms or reach the goal and drop exhausted into a batch of headache."[30] Graham agreed with Friedman that cluster headache arose because these patients suffered from a conflict between their external masculinity and internal passivity: "Behind their excessively manly fronts lie great dependency needs. They are led by the hand to the doctor's office often by the wife who takes the prescriptions, calls in the reports and makes the appointments."[31] Graham likened this behavior to a "mouse living inside a lion." This leonine exterior was written onto patients' bodies, which he described as having a rugged, masculine appearance, with a "ruddy complexion . . . multifurrowed, thick skin, [and] leonine facies."[32] Their skin was "peau d'orange," or pitted like the peel of an orange. Their overall portraits:

> present us with a picture of rugged, aggressive masculinity. The bodies that go with these faces are generally those of sturdy, muscular, mesomorphs. Athletic prowess is common. They tend to be a harder-drinking and harder-smoking lot than comparable groups of migraine subjects and controls. They are even more red-blooded males than any of their fellows. Over half of them have hemato-

> crits of 46 percent or over and quite a number range around 50 percent and some as high as 54 percent and 56 percent. And theirs is a male disease. In our series of 100 cluster patients, 90 are men, where as in a 100 common migraine patients only 30 are men. They tend, also, to have other diseases that belong chiefly to males.[33]

In these descriptions, Graham became the first physician to transform cluster headache from a condition that happens *to* men to a condition *of* men. His claim that patients share a physical manifestation of masculinity suggested some yet-to-be discovered underlying physiological cause of cluster headache—one that could also explain this excess in masculine appearance and behavior. This is also the first time that we see the metaphor of masculinity playing a strong role in the creation of medical knowledge of cluster headache. When Graham describes his patients as "red-blooded," he makes a metaphorical allusion to their virility. He backs up this claim with a reference to hematocrit levels (the proportion of blood that consists of packed red blood cells), proving that they are literally red-blooded.

Graham wrote that his female patients shared this masculine appearance. In the same 1972 article, he included four pictures of women with cluster headache, whom he described as having masculine features (see figure 5.1) The first, he says, has the classic "peau d'orange" skin. The second is "a very strong, powerful woman with a big frame and shoulders and arms and muscles"; the third looks "very much like the first woman"; while he describes the fourth woman as "a lady who comes from out West who's breaking broncos and running a ranch," adding, "I think you can see that her face presents the picture of a determined, rather masculine, square-faced powerful person." Graham preserves the feminine psyche behind the masculine physique: "In our experience, beneath their rather manly exterior these [women] patients have very sensitive female psyches and personality patterns."[34] Graham never specifies what is masculine about these women's appearances, other than their pitted skin and broad frames. But the pictures do not demonstrate this, nor do they explain why pitted skin and broad shoulders are masculine. Two of the women wear lipstick. Three appear older and wrinkled, which may be evidence of the characteristic leonine face. His ambiguity on the matter suggests that these descriptions were meant to be self-evident to the reader.

Graham and his theories proved influential. By 1976, he had been elected president of the American Association for the Study of Headache

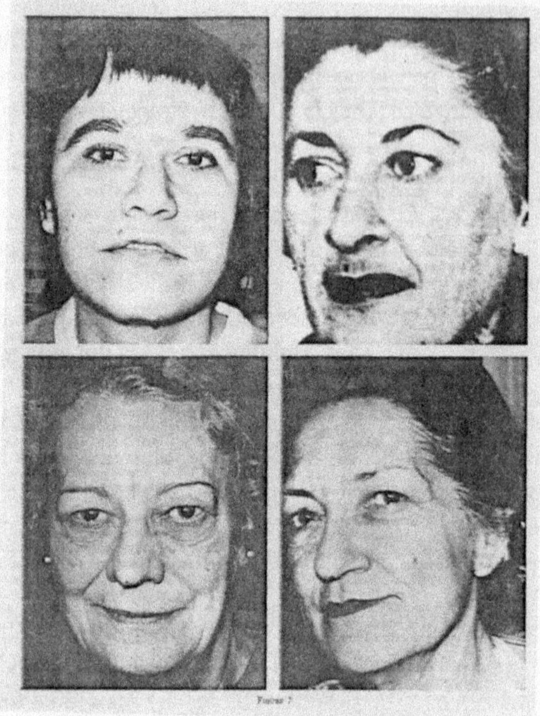

FIGURE 5.1 "Women with Cluster Headache," from Graham, John R. 1972. "Cluster Headache." *Headache* 11 (4): 175–85. Reprinted with permission from John Wiley and Sons.

(AASH). And his contributions to headache medicine continue to be recognized even today, notably by the American Headache Society (AHS), which has named one of its most coveted awards after him.

The Stubborn Persistence of the Cluster Profile

In the 1970s, Lee Kudrow produced a series of influential studies supporting Graham's cluster headache profile, particularly Graham's description of a leonine cluster headache physique. In one study based on twenty cluster headache patients and controls recruited from his headache clinic, Kudrow found that cluster patients tend to be taller, with a higher incidence of hazel eye color than control groups. (Kudrow shares these physical features.) He also concluded that "type A personality" features are common. Kudrow proposed a causal relationship between these factors, theorizing that the uptight personality of cluster patients led to heavy smoking and drinking, which then produced their characteristic leonine appearance.[35]

This research suffered from methodological flaws that were and continue to be overlooked in the headache literature. Much of it was based on exceedingly small samples—Kudrow analyzed as few as sixteen subjects. Moreover, he systematically excluded from analysis any subject who would counter particular findings; for example, black patients were left out of assessments of eye color and women were left out of the analysis of height and hemoglobin. Similarly, Kudrow developed rationales for excluding outliers. For example, "Only one man from the cluster group was shorter than 68 [inches]. He is a forty-six-year old Filipino, 65 [inches] tall."[36] Kudrow left out further explanation, but the implication was that the patient's Filipino ethnicity accounted for his short stature.

Kudrow did not, however, support Graham's psychodynamic assessment of the cluster patient as that of a "mouse inside a lion." He argued that such imagery pathologized what could be considered to be quite normal masculine characteristics: "It is neither unusual nor infrequently encountered that men, cluster or otherwise, take a subordinate position to their wives in respect to household mechanics and decisions which include doctors' appointments and the filling of prescriptions. It is not unlikely that wives of non-cluster males would have the same opinion of their husbands 'weaknesses' as wives of cluster males."[37] In other words, nothing could be more masculine than letting one's wife manage one's health care. In any case, if otherwise confident men shared their intimate fears and anxieties within the confines of a physician's office, it may not have been pathological as much as a normal expression of emotion caused by a painful, disruptive condition.

In later work, Kudrow and B. J. Sutkus tested the existence of a cluster headache personality, using the Minnesota Multiphasic Personality Inventory (MMPI), and found that both migraine and cluster headache patients have normal personalities.[38] Most subsequent studies using the MMPI and other personality tests have found little to no difference between cluster patients and controls.[39] A few studies have found elevated levels of "psychological disability" in cluster headache, but none have found differences between their cluster and migraine patients.[40] This work suggests that if migraine and cluster headache patients do have psychological problems, these problems are caused by pain, rather than the other way around.[41]

Few research studies have attempted to replicate Kudrow's findings in support of a cluster physique. Joel Saper, AHS president from 1990 to 1992, reported leonine facial features among the cluster patients in his clinic (as well as an inexplicable greater inclination for cluster patients to read gun magazines), but used no controls.[42] In 2000, a group calling itself the Italian Cooperative Study Group on the Epidemiology of Cluster Headache found no evidence of a cluster profile, with one exception: the cluster group had a slightly wider "mid-face height" than controls.[43] Nevertheless, two experts in the field were not able to identify cluster patients from case controls by physical appearance alone. This study raises questions about the cluster physique, but has received little attention in the medical literature.

There has also been a shift in the medical literature regarding the epidemiology of cluster headache. Many researchers are starting to believe that cluster headache may not be as male-dominated as once thought. Although early studies on cluster headache reported a male dominance of as much as nine or ten to one,[44] more recent studies have located more women with cluster headache, shifting the estimated gender ratio to two or three to one—a ratio that looks more like the demographic reverse of gender prevalence in migraine than the overwhelmingly male condition that cluster headache was once believed to be.[45]

Researchers' explanations for this shift illustrate just how deeply headache specialists are attached to thinking about cluster headache as a masculine problem. When, in 1998, research initially suggested that women may have cluster headache far more often than was previously believed, scholars were quick to attribute this finding to a true shift in epidemiology. Perhaps, they argued, "nontraditional" women were now more susceptible to cluster headache because they "acted" more like men by working, drinking, and smoking. This hypothesis alluded to a long-standing argument that men were predisposed to cluster headache due to a higher propensity toward injury to the hypothalamic-limbic center of the brain. Damage to the hypothalamus would explain the cyclic patterns of the disorder, since this is where the body controls its circadian and circannual rhythms. In addition, this argument made good use of studies that suggested that people with cluster headache were more likely to smoke cigarettes and drink alcohol.[46] Headache specialist Ottar Sjaastad added that "the male preponderance [of cluster headache] is associated with the role as *man* in modern society, irrespective of the sex hormones. The expectations to a man may be so high that it may be difficult for everybody to live up to them."[47] It is within this context that headache specialists like Gian Manzoni placed the blame on feminism, explaining that the increase in cluster headache in women is "a toll that women may have to pay for their liberation."[48] Authors of a 2001 review article agreed: "Cluster headache seems to be increasing in women, which may be secondary to women taking on the occupations and vices of men."[49] But just as this indictment of feminism conveniently forgets that women have always worked—if not always for pay—it also ignores the more obvious explanation for this rather dramatic shift in prevalence. Diagnostic practices have changed.

Evidence now suggests that doctors are more likely to apply the cluster headache diagnosis to women as they become more familiar with cluster headache symptoms and as doctors become more proficient in treating the disorder.[50] Evidence also suggests that cluster headache manifests itself differently in men and women. Women with cluster headache have symptoms that, at times, seem more migrainous. For example, when women with cluster headache report cluster-like pain (short-lived and intense), their pain is often accompanied by more migraine-like autonomic symptoms (nausea and light and sound sensitivity, rather than the usual cluster symptoms).[51] When these borderline cases are diagnosed as cluster headache, the gender ratio of the disorder changes.

The masculinized profile of cluster headache has remained remarkably persistent, even as researchers have redefined cluster headache as a neurovascular disorder, potentially involving the hypothalamus.[52] This is in stark contrast to migraine, for which headache specialists have used the new neurobiological paradigm to distance migraine from embarrassing psychosomatic theories of the past. Indeed, neurobiological theories of cluster headache are often found alongside psychosomatic characterizations of the cluster patient. Even though little evidence supports Graham's cluster headache profile, the profile continues to appear in medical textbooks. In order to uncover just how persistent this profile is, I conducted a content analysis of ninety-one reference books on headache, selected because they were available in the University of Michigan medical library, published between Graham's publication of the cluster profile in 1970 and 2005, and contained a nontrivial reference to cluster headache.[53]

Over the period under study, over half (53 percent) of medical textbooks that included a discussion of cluster headache also included a description of at least some of the features of the cluster profile. But, as one

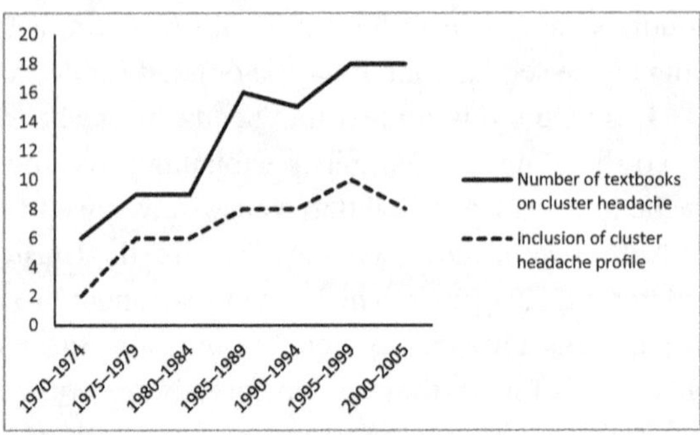

FIGURE 5.2 Persistence of cluster headache profile in textbooks.

might imagine, the coverage of cluster headache changed over time. First, over the years, the absolute number of books that include reference information on cluster headache increased. At the same time, the absolute number of books that include the cluster headache profile also increased, albeit more slowly. When the cluster profile was at its most popular (between 1975 and 1985), it was included in 67 percent of reference books. By 2000–2005, this rate dropped to 44 percent (see figure 5.2).

Authors were selective about which aspects of the profile they supported. Across all years, support for the cluster physique (82 percent) far exceeded support for the cluster psyche (28 percent). This differential support likely reflects the fact that far more research has investigated the existence of the cluster psyche than the existence of the cluster physique, and there is very little support in this literature in favor of a cluster psyche. On a few rare occasions, textbook authors included a description of the cluster profile with the sole purpose of rejecting it (usually as a myth, or as an obsolete idea). In these cases, authors were more likely to reject the cluster psyche (25 percent) than the cluster physique (13 percent). Overall, the cluster headache profile was more likely to appear in books written for a general medical audience (58 percent) or lay audience (46 percent) than in books written for an audience already expert in headache treatment (37 percent) (see figure 5.3).

One reason why the cluster profile might be so persistent is that its characterizations of men and women are not viewed as stigmatizing or problematic. Indeed, the cluster profile enjoys strong, if not unanimous, support from headache experts in the field. Headache specialists often evoked the cluster profile when presenting in professional research con-

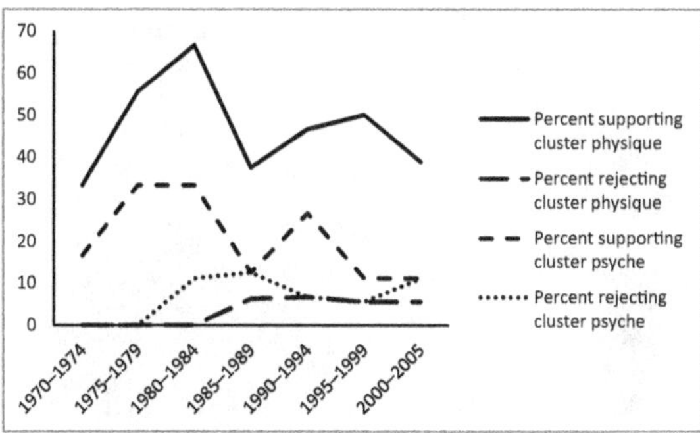

FIGURE 5.3 Percent of textbooks that support or reject the cluster profile.

ferences. Cluster patients were described as "somewhat dependent personalities, dependent on their wives—usually the wives tend to be the decision makers in the family. They tend to be rather large people, with wide faces, and peau d'orange skin" (fieldnotes). Even skeptical descriptions have the effect of perpetuating the cluster profile. For example, at a 2001 presentation of the Neurology Ambassador Program sponsored by the AHS and the American Academy of Neurology, David Dodick, a prominent cluster headache researcher, told a ballroom of more than a thousand attendees: "There have been a number of associated features of cluster headache . . . habits, phenotypic features—that many have said are more common in patients with cluster headache than in the general population[; for example,] the typical leonine faces, these heavy, coarse facial features, which we will not that infrequently see. . . . [We don't know] whether that's due to cluster headache, to [its] intrinsic nature . . . or whether that's due to the heavy tobacco use" (fieldnotes).

Dodick was careful not to endorse the leonine stereotype, preferring to use what scholars Ellen Prince, Joel Frader, and Charles L. Bosk call "hedging phrases."[54] By using phrases like "many have said" as opposed to a more accepting "studies have shown" and offering the counter explanation that tobacco causes leonine features, Dodick distanced himself from masculinized theories of cluster headache. Indeed, Dodick had discounted this profile in an article on cluster headache that he had published a year earlier.[55] Nevertheless, each of his PowerPoint slides was accompanied with an animated illustration of a typical cluster headache patient. In contrast to Dodick's rejection of the cluster headache profile, his slides represented the cluster headache patient face as leonine with hazel eyes.

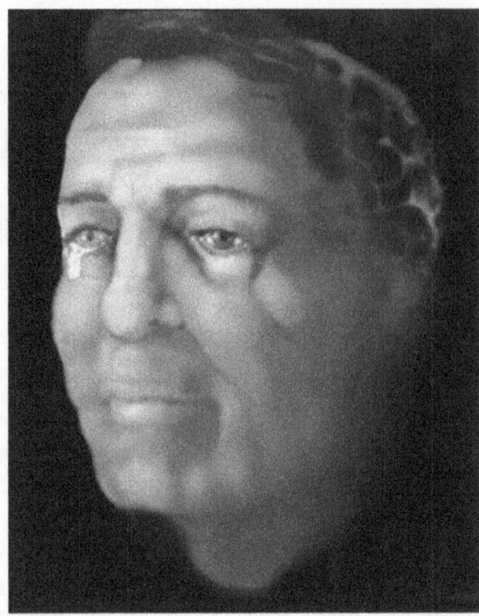

FIGURE 5.4 Typical representation of a cluster man. Cluster patient depicted in AAN's CME, *Brainstorm.*

The slides commit Dodick to the profile, no matter what his description (see figure 5.4.)

I found little evidence that the cluster profile received much critical attention in the field. One researcher told me that he collects images of cluster patients because he thinks it is "cool that they look so much like lions. Even the women look the same!" (fieldnotes). At the same time, other headache researchers told me that the cluster profile is a myth: "I don't know that I really can say that I've seen that [leonine face]. I mean, I look for it and every once in a while I see one and say, 'Oh, yeah, that guy is like that.' You know, sandy hair, hazel eyes, leonine creases, but I don't know that I really find that at all helpful in any way" (interview). These frequent encounters with the cluster profile demonstrate how ingrained these social, physical, and psychological images of cluster headache and masculinity are. It is important to keep in mind, however, that cluster headache is coded as masculine even in the absence of the cluster profile. For example, the cluster headache profile is *not* included in the opening description of cluster headache in which Alan Rapoport, Fred

Sheftell, and Stewart Tepper describe cluster headache as a pain so severe that it can topple even "the strongest of men." Thus, even as the cluster profile loses its hold on the headache community, its residual masculinity does not. The metaphorical connection between cluster headache and masculinity has grown so entrenched in the headache literature that these two ideas have melded into one unified concept. Consequently, when I asked headache specialists whether they thought it odd that cluster headache descriptions were so masculine, they often responded, "Cluster headache *is* masculine." But masculinity and femininity are culturally grounded, historically situated ideas. In lieu of research and debate about the relationship between gender and biology, medical researchers engage in a dangerous form of gender essentialism.

Cluster Headache and the Legitimacy Deficit

In previous chapters, I discussed how headache specialists frequently express concerns about a "courtesy stigma" that emerges from treating migraine patients. The same is not true for cluster headache. While doctors talk about the various ways in which they try to distance their profession from the public perception that their migraine patients have psychosomatic problems, no such similar discourse occurs with cluster headache, even though people with migraine and people with cluster headache are treated by the same doctors in the same clinics. To the contrary, headache specialists articulate a great deal of pride when working with cluster patients. Indeed, having a critical mass of cluster headache patients conveys status on a headache specialist. Part of this comes from the rarity of the disorder—only headache specialists from the most prestigious clinics have access to enough cluster patients to conduct research on this population. Part of this comes from the perceived severity of cluster headache. As David Dodick once said, "from a therapeutic standpoint, there's hardly anything more gratifying than those of us who look after headache patients to see a patient with cluster headache which is perhaps one of the most severe pains that one could possibly experience and to effectively treat that individual" (fieldnotes). But part of this attitude also comes from the moral characteristics associated with cluster headache. Treating a disorder known to "bring the strongest of men" to his knees has more appeal than treating a disorder associated with hysterical, sensitive women.

The masculinity associated with cluster headache, however, has not been sufficient to legitimate the experience of people who have cluster headache. In order to learn more about how people with cluster headache experience their disorder, I conducted a content analysis of an electronic support group that exists specifically for people with cluster headache. This analysis revealed that, like those with migraine, people who have cluster headache experience a legitimacy deficit—they have trouble getting a diagnosis, finding adequate health care, and communicating the severity of their illness to others. But unlike people who have migraine, people who have cluster headache are able to draw upon the masculinity embedded in their disorder as a resource in their efforts to legitimate their symptoms.

For example, people with cluster headache often complain that others do not understand their pain. Their frustrations are widespread, as evidenced by a discussion in an electronic support group that queried, "What's the dumbest thing someone's said to you when you're in cluster mode?" Answers ranged from "Stop eating cheese? Go to bed earlier? Just pull the curtains and have a wee lie down? Stop drinking those Red Bulls and you'll be alright?" to "Go back to your hotel, lay [*sic*] down, turn the lights off, take the phone off of the hook, and just relax! Hopefully that'll nip this in the bud!" to "You know what you need is two big shots of Jack [whiskey]" to "You just have too much stress in your life, stop worrying about stuff and give up coffee!" Others said that people thought that they were inventing their diagnosis: "It's all in your head" was a frequent refrain. One poster said that, almost thirty years earlier, he had been put into a psychiatric ward when a neurologist failed to recognize his pain as real. "The head neurologist came in and told me: "No one can have the pain you are '*pretending*' to have, without something showing up on the tests." Another complained: "Even some of the people I love think I'm inventing it, which makes me so angry. They've never run headlong to the fridge at 3am in the morning [*sic*] to find an egg to stick into your eye socket."

People with cluster headache also describe myriad encounters with disbelieving doctors and health care workers. One neurologist (not a headache specialist) reportedly told a cluster headache patient that "[cluster headache] happens only during spring and autumn. You can't have it all year. You must have psychological problems. You should see a therapist." Another wrote that when he was first in the hospital, a neurologist said, "Your scan is clear you haven't reacted to morphine so therefore the headaches are not real and you are depressed!" The emergency room is also fraught with delegitimizing experiences. People with cluster headache were sometimes mistaken for drug seekers, even though they requested oxygen, not pain medications. (Oxygen is a highly effective abortive for cluster headache.) In short, people with cluster headache describe "a medical system which has not effectively trained docs in treating Cluster. The same complaints are [repeatedly] posted here: poor diagnosis; inadequate treatment."

Posters often attribute the public's broad misunderstanding of cluster headache to a conflation with "headache" and/or "migraine." People report that others frequently respond to their cluster headaches by saying things like "yeah, I get headaches too" or "It's only a freaking headache—what's the big deal?" Conflation with migraine is just as disconcerting: "A friend has said 'yeah I get migraines too.'" Another reported that her employer responded to her cluster headaches by saying, "I get migraines too you just need to get at least eight hours of sleep." This piece of advice is particularly grating, since cluster headache often strikes people during their sleep, making sleep difficult and frightening.

Mistaking cluster headache for migraine or, worse, for headache, frustrates people with cluster headache because it suggests that others misunderstand the severity of cluster headache. These comparisons also raise highly gendered anxieties about how cluster headache pain is perceived. For example, one poster explained that the common misperception that cluster headache is akin to a headache bothers him: "'I've had that before' ticks me off. Being treated as though I'm just being a whimp [*sic*] over a 'headache.'" Since no one wants to be understood to be a "wimp," many people with cluster headache avoid describing their disorder using the word "headache." Says one poster, "I don't say cluster headaches. I say I have a malfunctioning brain." Others refer to cluster headaches as "attacks" or as "a rare neurological disorder." These strategies help distinguish cluster headache from more ordinary forms of head pain, but they also serve to distance cluster headache from the highly feminized characteristics associated with migraine. As one poster put it, "We don't say headaches or migraines. We're like 'He has a brain disease.' People shut up. It's just easier. We used to say 'Wicked headaches' but people just think he is a sissy that can't handle a migraine." Neurobiology, here, is called upon as a resource to resist interpretations that people with cluster headache are "sissies"—another feminized attack.

This isn't to say that people with cluster headache unquestioningly embrace the highly masculinized cluster profile. In fact, most patient advocacy groups have long since disregarded it as an untenable stereotype. Bill Pahlow, founder of OUCH, told me: "We (at OUCH) poo-poo that. We kind of write that off as old school stuff. You know, they say they're [people with cluster headache] big men with, you know, square jaws and orange peel skin. Usually being led into the office by a petite wife, a small wife. Um . . . we don't see that a whole lot in the people in our organization." Indeed, the general consensus across cluster headache advocacy groups seems to be that the gender ratio of cluster headache is much less male dominated than medical researchers think. Advocates who post about the stereotype often make fun of it. In the following passage, posted on clusterheadaches.com, the author teases researchers: "Epidemiological studies are even used to describe [us] in such specific terms as to make the whole idea of research laughable. Like, they're all male (loada crap—we LOVE female fans!), hazel-eyed (that one really slays me), bad complexioned (that one's sort of offensive), twenty-something (we do NOT discriminate on the basis of age) drunken smokers." DJ, the founder of clusterheadaches.com, combatted these stereotypes with an online survey that assessed the traits of people with cluster headache who came to his site for help. While acknowledging that his survey could not meet "scientific" standards, DJ told me that the findings were revealing.[56] The survey ended January 10, 2013, and found only 68 percent of the respondents reported that they were male, resulting in a gender ratio of about two to one. Nor does the survey support Graham's cluster profile: only 19 percent of respondents reported that they had hazel eyes, whereas 33 percent reported brown eyes and 32 percent reported blue eyes. In addition, almost half (48 percent) of the respondents reported that they were nonsmokers. DJ told me that

> the stuff that always bothered us was, you know, several years ago, here's what a cluster sufferer was, and if you weren't a man, and if you didn't have orange-peel skin, and you weren't a heavy drinker and a heavy smoker, it couldn't be cluster headache. I think a lot of that has gone. I think it might say, sure, if you are a heavy drinker and a heavy smoker it might make it worse, but it's not so cut and dry as it was before. And it came from the women, to be honest with you, because women were saying, I know for a fact that I have cluster headaches, but this criteria says I don't. So, their doctors just go, oh you're a woman, you can't have them.

At the same time, people with cluster headache experience some advantages of the highly masculinized profile associated with cluster headache. Pahlow, for example, admits that he enjoys the reputation that cluster headache has for being masculine and tough. On the message board of OUCH, he thinks that the men sometimes claim cluster headache for themselves, deriding the women who have the condition:

BP: But the men do get kind of possessive, you know, I mean I always see posts on the message board kind of half tongue in cheek saying, you know, women don't get clusters. You know, it's a male disease.

JK: Do you think they don't want to be associated with something that's female, you know what I mean? Like migraines have this sort of image about them.

BP: Yeah. Um . . . speaking as a male, I wouldn't [laughs]. To be totally honest with you. Even though everything I read says that cluster pain is worse than migraine pain, I think I'd rather have clusters than migraines because clusters are seen as a male disease. Versus migraines, which you really acquaint with a female disease.

Pahlow's confession reveals ambivalence regarding the masculinity associated with cluster headache. On one hand, the cluster profile fails to describe many people with cluster headache. On the other, there's a certain admiration that can accompany the masculinity associated with cluster headache. Cluster headache conveys toughness and resilience. Masculinity can be used to distinguish cluster headache from more feminized—and lower status—disorders like migraine.

Masculinity as a Source of Status and Legitimacy in Medicine

Virtually from its inception in the medical literature, physicians have understood cluster headache to be a disorder predominant in men. Eventually, this basic epidemiological association evolved into the framing of cluster headache as a disorder of excess masculinity. The stereotypical portrayal of cluster patients—as rugged, athletic men—suggests that the problem has something to do with a biological propensity toward masculinity. But the masculinity described in this literature is drawn from idealized western norms regarding hegemonic masculinity, not some innate or universal feature of men.[57]

The language used to describe cluster headache illustrates just how feminized our understanding of migraine is. Both disorders are tremendously painful, but migraine is characterized by retreat and described as a disorder of feminized sensitivity—the brain is hypersensitive to stimuli—while cluster headache is characterized as violent and aggressive and described as a disorder of masculinity—caused by risk taking and resulting in a condition marked by hyperrrational (alarm clock) pain. But these characterizations aren't inevitable, or even obvious, representations of the biology of migraine and cluster headache. People with migraine may want to retreat, but frequently cannot. They must continue working or caring for their children. Meanwhile, people with cluster headache describe how they must retreat when they have an attack, no matter what it is they are doing. Cluster headache is simply too painful to continue working during an attack. Migraine has its own cycles: many people regularly have their migraines upon waking (possibly triggered by REM sleep), or monthly (triggered by menstrual cycles), but these cycles are never described as rational. Meanwhile, many people with cluster headache argue that there is no rhythm to their cluster attacks.

The enduring presence of masculinity in the cluster headache literature also raises a number of questions about the relationship between representation of disease, the production of medical knowledge, and the legitimacy deficit. Clearly, cluster headache suffers from a legitimacy deficit, particularly when it comes to NIH's paltry funding of research on the disorder. This analysis suggests that, within headache medicine, the legitimacy deficit is smaller for cluster headache than for migraine, in large part because cluster headache is masculine. Headache doctors embrace the hypermasculinized cluster profile, even though little evidence supports it. The same might be said about people with cluster headache. Although they clearly experience a legitimacy deficit, their worries are that their head pain will be confused for highly feminized forms of headache—that is, that they will be taken for a wimp or a sissy. Indeed, physicians and some patients *admire* the cluster personality. The masculine characteristics associated with cluster headache—strength, stoicism, athleticism, rugged looks, and behavior—are *valued* at the same time that they are pathologized. The cluster profile suggests strength and vigor, not the psychological weakness associated with pain conditions. Cluster's masculine rhetoric confers status on both patients and physicians—patients because they are viewed as strong individuals experiencing serious and important pain and physician-specialists because a masculinized disorder can only heighten the status of their subject. That the masculinity of cluster headache raises the disorder's status stands in direct contrast to women's disorders, which are so often ignored, delegitimized, and dismissed. Masculinity, in this context, becomes a resource from which researchers and patients may draw in order to gain status and legitimacy. The payoff is significant and real.

These benefits may help explain how the extraordinary assumptions about masculinity remained embedded within cluster headache for so long. Indeed, it seems that a masculinized discourse inspires no natural critics. Even those opposed to hegemonic masculinity are not likely to critique its medicalization. Critics of hegemonic masculinity have long argued that masculinity is dangerous to both sexes, by encouraging unnecessary risk taking, exposing men to more occupational hazards, and burdening men with stresses caused by their traditional "breadwinning" role.[58] Because these scholars have already tried to pathologize masculinity, they are unlikely to be troubled by any attempts of medicine to further pathologize masculinity. The social construction of masculinity as a risky, oppressive attribute is typically forwarded as a progressive strand of gender theorizing, one that takes a stand against patriarchal power. Thus, the medicalization of masculinity has supporters from across the political spectrum: from those who privilege traditional masculinity to those who abhor it.

The persistence of this masculine discourse must be understood as the natural consequence of everyday thinking in medicine and what Ludwig Fleck called "the self contained" nature of scientific thought. As he described it, "the interaction between what is already known, what remains to be learned, and those who are to apprehend it, go to ensure harmony within the system."[59] In other words, cultural stereotypes may be more resilient than the emergence of new biological knowledge.

In some respects, feminist scholars have been successful in transforming the cultural stereotypes of women in medicine, inspiring what Steven Epstein terms "a new common sense" about how research on women and medicine ought to be conducted and interpreted.[60] Once acceptable research methods and interpretations now appear absurd and unethical. By sensitizing social scientists to subtle forms of gender inequality embedded within medical research, feminists have provided researchers with a different framework for interpreting their data, allowing for the emergence of new biological understandings of sex and gender. Yet, as migraine and cluster headache show, assumptions about masculinity and femininity remain deeply embedded within the language of these disorders. Migraine and cluster headache demonstrate that even researchers who are highly attuned to criticisms of sexism can end up reproducing and reifying the same gendered assumptions about their patients that they are trying to avoid. Gender is persistent; even as we try to alter power relations in medicine, the universal patient is embedded within a broader sociocultural gender system that promotes gender essentialism in medicine.

Conclusion

The Republican Party struggled to find a strong candidate to run against Barack Obama in the 2012 presidential elections. Former Massachusetts governor Mitt Romney, an early favorite, faced many challengers, including Representative Michele Bachmann, a conservative congresswoman who, with the backing of the so-called Tea Party movement, had won the Ames, Iowa, straw poll. But her candidacy took a major hit when on July 18 of that year, the *Daily Caller*, a conservative website, reported that she had migraine.

The article, headlined "Stress-Related Condition 'Incapacitates' Bachmann; Heavy Pill Use Alleged," featured quotes from several of Bachmann's former congressional staffers who argued that Bachmann couldn't handle the stress of the presidency, as she spent several hours, if not days, of each week in a darkened room, gripped by migraine symptoms. The article portrayed her as a "pill-popper" who wilted when confronted with even the smallest stresses. One aide claimed that Bachmann had responded to the resignation of a trusted staffer by developing a migraine so debilitating that she wound up in the hospital. An advisor said, "She carries and takes all sorts of pills. Prevention pills. Pills during the migraine. Pills after the migraine, to keep them under control. She has to take these pills wherever she goes." In what could not be characterized as a slow news week (the country was absorbed by a political crisis about lifting the debt ceiling), Bachmann's migraine story received an enormous amount of interest. Bachmann verified that she had migraine, but vehemently denied that the condition was incapacitating, arguing that she managed her migraines with medication and that they would not affect her ability to function as president.

Journalists, headache advocates, doctors, and pundits agreed that the

Daily Caller's story was unnecessarily inflammatory—most thought that the headline was designed to incite opposition to Bachmann; that the article, which used only anonymous sources, read like a smear; and that charges of heavy drug use mischaracterized what was probably normal medical management of migraine. Commentators on the left uncharacteristically jumped to Bachmann's defense, criticizing media portrayals of Bachmann as sexist. They pointed, for example, toward the widely reported allegation that Bachmann, herself, attributed her migraines to wearing high-heel shoes. The ensuing debate outraged headache advocates, who read the media frenzy as indicative of the stigma associated with migraine. They particularly took issue with the characterization of migraine as a "stress-related condition," a phrase that seemed to draw on historical representations of people with migraine as hysterical, neurotic women. Instead, they asked the media to report the "truth that Migraine is a neurological disease."[1] Bachmann, they said, isn't a weak woman who "pops pills" and wouldn't be able to handle the stress of the presidency; she's a person who has a disease as real as diabetes and, like a diabetic, requires medication to manage her disorder. The public merely needed education on this new fact.

But much of the reporting on Bachmann *did* refer to migraine as neurobiological. Some of the online articles even linked to videos or animated pictures of the brain so that readers could see what really "causes" migraine. These references, however, did surprisingly little to temper the rendering of Bachmann's character as hysterical. Even articles that explicitly referred to migraine as neurobiological tended to describe Bachmann as hysterical. For example, in a July 20, 2011, article, the online news site *Politico* reported migraine as a serious neurobiological disease but added stigmatizing details such as the following: "The condition affects her brain and requires her to take psychoactive drugs" (even though they had no idea what kind of drugs she took) and "This is an issue that is neurological in nature, that affects consciousness and the ability to think clearly."

These sorts of comments managed simultaneously to acknowledge that migraine is biologically based and to suggest that the disease compromised Bachmann's rationality. Neurobiological language—when it found its way into media stories—merely traded the stigma of hysteria for a more resilient, reified stigma of irrationality. Bachmann's story illustrated the contradictory and vexed nature of contemporary public discourse on migraine. It is as likely that migraine will be represented as trivial (e.g., caused by wearing high heels) as it is to be represented as severe (e.g., affecting consciousness). Either way, the introduction of neurobiology as a cause of migraine has done little to clarify public understanding of the diagnosis or to squelch hyper-gendered representations of the disorder.

Neurobiology and the Legitimacy Deficit

To understand why the neurobiological turn in migraine has done little to improve the public's perception of migraine as a legitimate disease, it helps to recognize that a given disease's acceptance as "legitimate" is not a simple process: it involves multiple dimensions that may not be fully attained at once. Migraine offers a good vantage point for understanding the layers involved in establishing both the reality and the cultural status of a disease. As an invisible disease, its ontology has to be established at both the biological level (i.e., does migraine as a disease exist?) and at an individual level (i.e., does this specific person have a migraine when she says that she does?), and at a cultural level (i.e., is this diagnosis serious and deserving of resources?). The case of migraine shows legitimacy depends on much more than medical agreement of diagnostic criteria: even though its existence as a "real" medical disorder has been established, individual patients continue to have difficulty convincing their doctors both that they have it and that their symptoms are serious. And even medical acceptance, should it be obtained, is not sufficient to convince friends, family, coworkers, and employers of the severity of the disease. Thus, the legitimation of migraine takes on a moral dimension, as people who have it must prove that they are reliable reporters of their symptoms. Most stakeholders in the headache community have addressed this by focusing their attention on proving that migraine is a "real neurobiological disease," forgetting that this is only half the battle. It hardly matters if migraine is established as a specific disease if individual patients are not believed or, if when they are, they are not thought to have a serious disorder.

Migraine's status is complicated by the fact that it has long been understood to be a diagnosis that affects a person with particular moral qualities—a neurotic, feminized character who cannot withstand the stresses of everyday life. This characterization, at least in part, reflects the epidemiology of migraine; migraines *are* more common in women than in men. But it is troubling to see the way that this epidemiological difference has been encoded into medical knowledge. Whether male or female, doctors have portrayed the typical migraine patient as hypersensitive and highly attuned to his or her environment. In previous eras, doctors believed that this sensibility came with advantages, for example, increased intelligence and artistry. Men with migraine were often depicted as studious and hardworking, if a bit passive. Women, on the other hand, were portrayed in a more negative light, typically as behaving in ways that breached their proper social roles or that avoided their expected duties. Patients of both sexes were thought to come from the upper classes; migraine was a lifestyle condition that affected those who had sensitive nervous systems. Working-class folk, who had thicker, ropier nerves, were made of stronger stuff.

Against this backdrop, imagining migraine as a disease of the brain seems positively radical. Foregrounding the brain as the problem drops the problematic patient out of view. The brain, in contrast to the patient, is a blank slate; unlike pesky individuals, complicated by problems of personality and subjectivity, the brain is constituted by neurons that merely fire on and off. By this logic, a neurobiological framework might remove some of the blame from headache patients: if migraine is a disease of the brain, then headache patients ought not be held responsible for their pain.

Headache specialists like this reframing. For centuries, doctors with an interest in treating headache disorders have complained of low status and low pay. But neurobiology made them optimistic. Indeed, headache specialists' embrace of the brain as a cause of migraine is as much symbolic as it is scientific. It distances them from their predecessors who, they argue, too readily attributed migraine to women's weak minds. The brain, they believe, not only holds the answers to migraine causation and prevention, but can also attract much-needed and desired financial resources from the pharmaceutical industry and the National Institutes of Health. In short, the brain offers the best available option to improve their profession's status.

And indeed, in some important ways, neurobiology has bolstered claims that migraine and cluster headache are specific diseases that ought to be treated by health care professionals. For example, when neurologists in headache medicine sought to redefine migraine as a neurobiological phenomenon, the first thing they did was to reconceptualize and strengthen the diagnostic criteria for migraine. Although migraine previously fell within medicine's jurisdiction, it was not well defined; the uniformity offered by these new diagnostic criteria suggested universality of the migraine experience. Likewise, fMRIs of migraines in progress provide visual evidence that migraine is rooted in the brain. In turn, neurobiology strengthened headache medicine as a specialty. Although headache specialists still complain that they "get no respect," their status has improved somewhat since their embrace of neurobiology. For one thing, they now have board certification from the American Academy of Neurology. Attention to the brain has also won them a strong alliance with the pharmaceutical industry. The two most promising developments in headache treatment both target the brain. Drug makers are testing calcitonin gene related peptide (CGRP) receptor antagonists that would provide a novel treatment to abort migraines, as well as neurostimulators that use electrical currents to activate or modulate neurons. The brain, a symbol of technological sophistication, points the way toward a better and brighter future for those who have migraine.

Not surprisingly, many people who have migraine are excited about the neurobiological paradigm, not only for the promise of new therapies, but also for the potential it has to legitimate their experiences. People with migraine share devastating stories in online communities; they describe the various ways that family, friends, employers, doctors, and bureaucracies fail to recognize how pervasive and serious their symptoms are. They struggle with the gap between a public that views them as having "just a headache," and a private reality in which migraine confines them to their houses and makes them unable to accomplish even the most basic tasks. The neurobiological paradigm for migraine offers an appealing portrayal of their symptoms; the notion of a "brain disease" captures the severity of symptoms that, in many cases, have taken over their lives. But beyond having their disease taken seriously, this embodied health movement hopes that a neurobiological model of migraine can help divest individuals of responsibility for their illness and free them from the implication that their disorder is psychological. They are tired of being told their symptoms would be better "if only they would relax" or that they should just "focus on something else." The brain, they hope, will transform migraine from something that exists "all in their mind" to a disease that is rooted in their brain. In short, both doctors and patients view the brain as a salve to historical constructions of migraine as affecting neurotic, hysterical characters incapable of withstanding the stresses of everyday life.

The problem, I have argued, is that the neurobiological paradigm hews too closely to personhood. Although social scientists have traditionally posited a straightforward relationship between specific disease mechanisms and legitimation, the brain may be an exceptional body part. The brain is the organ of subjectivity and personhood in the West. We are becoming, according to sociologists Francisco Ortega and Fernando Vidal, "cerebral subjects," increasingly defining ourselves by our brains, rather than by our minds.[2] So while a neurobiological frame may be able to root migraine in a biological process, it is a biological process that is closely associated with what makes us human. Brain explanations may be less able to separate disease from personhood than diseases stemming from other organs. Treating the brain as simply a body part "like any other" is anachronistic in an era when science and technology are teaching us that qualities like thought, behavior, rationality, will, and identity are neurobiological processes, rather than transcendental products of the mind. As a result, locating an illness in the brain might not be as legitimating as attributing an illness to the breakdown of another body part, like the stomach, or to inflammation of a tendon. It might, in fact, be perceived as a disorder of personhood—much as psychosomatic disorders were understood in the mid-twentieth century. Perhaps this is why we can see characteristics like hypersensitivity carrying over from psychosomatic medicine into neurobiological explanations of migraine. The brain may be more prone to moralizing discourses than other parts of the body.

"Brain blame" is unlikely to transform the moral characteristics associated with migraine patients. If, in the psychosomatic era, people with migraine were thought to be a particular kind of person, that is, hypersensitive, neurotic, and weak, it is not clear that all that much has changed under the neurobiological paradigm. The primary difference is that now people with migraine are thought to have brains that are hypersensitive, neurotic, and weak. The hypersensitive neurons that constitute the migraine brain tell the same story about migraine patients that Harold G. Wolff told in the mid-twentieth century, albeit using the brain, rather than the vascular system. The moral character of the migraine patient has been encoded directly into the biological body. The neurobiological paradigm doesn't clear the deck of gendered personhood; at best it merely shuffles the chairs.

In any case, the problem with migraine has never been that doctors failed to recognize it as a biological phenomenon. Since Galen, physicians have located migraine in the body, whether they thought the problem was a humoral imbalance, a structural disruption in the brain, a stomach disturbance, an inherited sensitivity of the nervous system, or a volatile vascular system. Indeed, doctors always understood the symptoms and pain of migraine to be physical; more questionable was the moral character associated with people who experienced this pain. Doctors wrote about people with migraine as characters who thought too hard or wrongly;

obsessed too much or who worried about the wrong things; whose passions raged—unless, that is, the problem was that they were repressed. The body, in these older formulations, responded to emotional and psychological pressures by having migraines. The neurobiological paradigm revolutionized this model not by cleansing the migraine patient of moral character but by embodying it. Consequently, the identification of a specific biological mechanism for disease, by providing a strong epistemological account of its reality, provides only one dimension of legitimation. The neurobiological paradigm does little to provide for another dimension of legitimation—an improved moral character associated with the patient.

Gender and the Legitimacy Deficit

What makes the idea of a hysteric, neurotic woman or a strong, stoic man so compelling that it gets reinscribed into the body by researchers and doctors, accepted and even embraced by activists, and commodified, packaged, and disseminated by corporations? In other words, why are gendered categories of personhood so *persistent*, to the point that they have been inscribed into the brain?

The persistence of gender categories is a perennial puzzle for feminist scholars who have tried to explain the resilience of a hierarchical gender system, given that the world has changed in ways that ought to promote a more equal distribution of power. This book provides strong support for the argument that societal patterns of gender inequality are enacted through the endemic use of gender as a framing device for organizing thoughts about the body.[3] That is, even as the neurobiological paradigm transformed how headache specialists understand the onset and duration of migraine and cluster headache, sex and gender remain primary frames guiding "who" doctors, advocates, and marketers think of as having headache disorders. These cultural notions then get repurposed in surprising ways, even influencing scientific research that was initiated to counter gender stereotypes.

Behind the seemingly gender-neutral brain lie hundreds of waiting rooms and electronic support groups filled with white, middle-class female migraine patients and, to a lesser extent, white, male cluster headache patients. These spaces make it difficult for doctors, advocates, and advertisers to "see" the empirical reality of who has headache disorders in the population. Contrary to claims that migraine "just is a disorder of women" or that cluster headache "just *is* more masculine," headache patients are a diverse group. Six percent of US adult men have migraine, a number that constitutes one-quarter of all of those who have the diagnosis. African-Americans have migraine at nearly the same rate as whites and the prevalence of migraine increases significantly at lower income levels. This diversity, however, is almost completely absent from discourse about migraine. At first, this diversity gets filtered out at the doctor's office. Headache specialists are difficult to access—few doctors are board certified to practice headache medicine, meaning that it often takes many referrals, persistence, and a significant amount of money to get an appointment. (When my own headache doctor accepts new headache patients, a rare occurrence, he screens them for mental illness, which includes taking a rather expensive personality test and meeting with a psychiatrist and a psychologist, neither of whom accept insurance payments.) As a result, only those with the best insurance and some disposable income are likely to make it through the system. Men also have a difficult time getting this care, as they are less likely to seek help for head pain and, when they do go to the clinic, they are less likely to receive a diagnosis of migraine.[4] A similar gender discrepancy occurs in the case of cluster headache. However, it is men who are more likely to receive this diagnosis.[5] The situation is even more difficult for cluster headache, given that even some headache specialists are ill prepared to treat it.

But the story doesn't end in the clinic. The presumption that migraine is a women's disease and that cluster headache is a men's disease has become so intrinsic to thought about headache disorders that it has spread across contexts, infusing everything that doctors, advocates, and the pharmaceutical industry purport to know about migraine and cluster headache. Migraine is thus described in classically feminine terms: the person with migraine is hypersensitive to the environment and retreats into a dark, quiet room to handle pain in the most passive of ways. Even when the patient is not having symptoms, he or she is described as having an almost superhuman capacity for intuition, a capability that is traditionally understood to be feminine. The cluster patient, in contrast, responds to pain in an aggressive fashion, pacing and rocking, pulling on hair and pushing into skin. The cluster patient's pain behaves in a rational way, occurring with the regularity of a clock. Cluster headache asserts itself and is insensitive to external triggers. The migraine patient hides; the cluster patient fights.

What's more, the pharmaceutical industry, whose products are often credited with ushering in the neurobiological paradigm, is one of the most prolific purveyors of this highly gendered vision of migraine. Migraine advertisements uniformly depict migraine as a minor disorder that mostly just gets in the way of how white middle-class women like to live their life. The gender dynamics of these advertisements evoke a psychosomatic era that portrayed women as simpering, fragile beings, hands pressed to their foreheads, forced to lie down on chaise longues. In the modern version, women are shown as having more responsibilities, albeit ones that they cannot fulfill. A typical contemporary migraine ad shows a woman being kept from carework—a fate made clear because she is ignoring a child while her hand is pressed up against her forehead. These advertisements trade in a highly stereotyped version of womanhood that is both easily recognizable and, presumably, easy to identify with. The net result is the propagation of more images that connect migraine with cultural notions of weak femininity.

Gender also continues to pose problems for people who have migraine and cluster headache, according to their accounts posted online. And yet, the same people who revile the commonplace understanding of migraine as a problem limited to hysterical women are perfectly happy to accept neurobiological accounts of migraine as a disease of hypersensitive brains. Indeed, advocates accept normative prescriptions of gender, as long as they are confined to their brains—despite the fact that these descriptions continue to limit how people with migraine are understood. I was less surprised to learn that cluster headache advocates embraced the masculinity of their diagnosis. Whereas legitimation strategies for people with migraine hinge on distinguishing between the real and unreal, cluster patients' strategies often depend on creating distance between a masculine cluster headache and a feminized migraine diagnosis (i.e, in proving that cluster headache is *not* migraine). In their logic, migraine equals feminine equals unreal; hence the ontological route they take must pass through the masculine. This means that their explanations of cluster headache also pass through the brain (as they explain, they have a terrible brain disease).

The brain, however, is anything but gender neutral—in this case, it serves as a tabula rasa, absorbing and reifying assumptions about gender. Neuroscience has quietly created a revolution in how we understand how we relate to others, how our brains relate to our bodies, and how we understand our selves. Neuroimaging, psychopharmaceuticals that can change mood and enhance memory and attention, brain stimulation devices, and neuroenhancement technologies are providing new ways of understanding and intervening in our brains. This book demonstrates that gender still matters in the framing of neurobiological *disease*. The question is, how will neurobiological *technologies* alter gender relations? Will new insights into the workings of the brain challenge gender hierarchies? Or will they serve to further solidify power relations around race, class, and gender?

Advocacy and the Legitimacy Deficit

Despite the obvious role of gender in maintaining the legitimacy deficit in both migraine and cluster headache, it feels strange to blame gender for the problems facing headache disorders in an era when other women's diseases are thriving in the political realm. At least, this is the complaint leveled at me every time I present my findings to headache specialists and advocates. How is it, these critics ask, that gender contributes to the marginalization of headache disorders when breast cancer, once a highly stigmatized disease, is now one of the best funded, most discussed diagnoses in the United States?

Here, I think it is important to keep three things in mind. First, the diagnosis of breast cancer depends on technologies like mammogram and biopsy that make the disease visible. Unlike migraine, diagnosis of breast cancer is *not* dependent on the subjective reporting of the patient. Indeed, many women have no idea that they have breast cancer until they receive the diagnosis from their doctor. Power relations, here, reside squarely with the doctor. Second, body parts matter in the legitimation of disease. Women's breasts—symbols of love, femininity, sexuality, motherhood, and eroticism—are valued differently in a patriarchal society than women's brains, which are the seat of (ir)rationality, personality, and character. The idea that society ought to safeguard and maintain women's breasts may be more easily embraced than the parallel notion that women's brains require the same sort of protection. Third, and perhaps most importantly, breast cancer receives so much funding because it was the subject of a highly successful social movement. Breast cancer is not the norm; it is an outlier that receives a disproportionately high level of funding given its relative burden on society.[6]

There are nevertheless lessons to be learned from looking closely at breast cancer advocacy's success as a social movement. Disease advocacy can and does lead to direct increases in research funding.[7] Here, headache disorders have been at a huge disadvantage relative to other diseases because, until very recently, advocates made little effort to lobby the federal government to increase research funds and resources for headache medicine. However, this is starting to change. Every year since 2007, a headache-specialist-led organization called the Alliance for Headache Disorders Advocacy (AHDA) has arranged for patients, advocates, and representatives from a variety of different headache organizations to travel to Washington, DC, to meet with congressional staff. During visits, headache advocates present their members of Congress with a long list of requests. Recent requests include language that would direct the National Institutes of Health (NIH) to increase funding for research and training in headache medicine, to include chronic migraine among the list of diseases funded by the Department of Defense's Congressional Directed Medical Research Program, to initiate a congressional hearing on headache disorders, and to encourage members of Congress to write a letter of support to the Social Security Administration that migraine be included as a category of disability. Many of these requests have already been fulfilled, leading to millions of dollars of additional funding. These efforts have already demonstrated some success and ought to be supported and enlarged.

However, to be truly successful, headache advocates must directly address the moral judgments so often made about the character of those who have headache disorders. This is as true at the policy level as it is at the interpersonal level. The stigma associated with migraine contributes to the legitimacy deficit, eroding the identity of the person with migraine, harming her ability to seek and receive care, and embedding itself into institutional policies created about people in pain. As sociologist Rachel Kahn Best has discovered, disease advocacy has had the unintended consequence of making moral character increasingly relevant to decisions about disease funding. Rather than arguing that funding decisions should be based on scientific proposals (thus making the disease or the scientist the beneficiary of grants), disease advocates have encouraged policy makers to think of *patients* as beneficiaries of research dollars. The end result has been a funding system in which nonstigmatized diseases that affect populations who appear deserving have a clear advantage over stigmatized diseases that affect populations that appear undeserving.[8]

How ought headache advocates go about removing the stigma of migraine and cluster headache? If neurobiology can't save headache disorders, what hope is there for people in pain? As a person with chronic migraine, these are the questions that worry me the most. One possibility is to stop focusing on etiology. Perhaps there's no use in trying to convince people that headache disorders are real. Maybe, instead, we should focus attention on reframing stories about the people who have headache disorders. If I've learned anything over the course of my research, it's that people with headache disorders are everywhere, and they aren't the hysterical neurotic whiners of popular culture. Quite the contrary: it takes great strength and stamina to live and work with a headache disorder. People with headache disorders are fighters. They struggle, but they survive and very often they thrive, despite enormous pain and disability.

Appendix A

International Classification of Headache Disorders
(3rd edition, beta version)
1. Migraine without aura
Previously used terms:
Common migraine; hemicrania simplex.
Description:
Recurrent headache disorder manifesting in attacks lasting 4–72 hours. Typical characteristics of the headache are unilateral location, pulsating quality, moderate or severe intensity, aggravation by routine physical activity and association with nausea and/or photophobia and phonophobia.
Diagnostic criteria:

A. At least 5 attacks fulfilling criteria B–D
B. Headache attacks lasting 4–72 hours (untreated or unsuccessfully treated)
C. Headache has at least 2 of the following characteristics:
    1. unilateral location
    2. pulsating quality
    3. moderate or severe pain intensity
    4. aggravation by or causing avoidance of routine physical activity (*eg*, walking or climbing stairs)
D. During headache at least 1 of the following:
    1. nausea and/or vomiting
    2. photophobia and phonophobia
E. Not better accounted for by another ICHD-3 diagnosis

1.2 Migraine with aura

Previously used terms:

Classic or classical migraine; ophthalmic, hemiparaesthetic, hemiplegic or aphasic migraine; migraine accompagne; complicated migraine.

Description:

Recurrent attacks, lasting minutes, of unilateral fully reversible visual, sensory or other central nervous system symptoms that usually develop gradually and are usually followed by headache and associated migraine symptoms.

Diagnostic criteria:

A. At least two attacks fulfilling criteria B and C
B. One or more of the following fully reversible aura symptoms:
   1. visual
   2. sensory
   3. speech and/or language
   4. motor
   5. brainstem
   6. retinal
C. At least two of the following four characteristics:
   1. at least one aura symptom spreads gradually over 5 minutes, and/or two or more symptoms occur in succession
   2. each individual aura symptom lasts 5–60 minutes
   3. at least one aura symptom is unilateral
   4. the aura is accompanied, or followed within 60 minutes, by headache
D. Not better accounted for by another ICHD-3 diagnosis, and transient ischaemic attack has been excluded.

1.3 Chronic migraine

Description:

Headache occurring on 15 or more days per month for more than 3 months, which has the features of migraine headache on at least 8 days per month.

Diagnostic criteria:

A. Headache (tension-type-like and/or migraine-like) on 15 days per month for >3 months and fulfilling criteria B and C

B. Occurring in a patient who has had at least five attacks fulfilling criteria B–D for 1.1 Migraine without aura and/or criteria B and C for 1.2 Migraine with aura
C. On ≥8 days per month for >3 months, fulfilling any of the following 3:
   1. criteria C and D for 1.1 Migraine without aura
   2. criteria B and C for 1.2 Migraine with aura
   3. believed by the patient to be migraine at onset and relieved by a triptan or ergot derivative
D. Not better accounted for by another ICHD-3 diagnosis.

3. Cluster headache and other trigeminal autonomic cephalalgias
3.1 Cluster headache
Previously used terms:
Ciliary neuralgia; erythro-melalgia of the head; erythroprosopalgia of Bing; hemicranias angioparalytica; hemicranias neuralgiformis chronica; histaminic cephalalgia; Horton's headache; Harris-Horton's disease; migrainous neuralgia (of Harris); petrosal neuralgia (of Gardner); Sluder's neuralgia; spheno-palatine neuralgia; vidian neuralgia.
Coded elsewhere:
Symptomatic cluster headache, secondary to another disorder, is coded as a secondary headache attributed to that disorder.
Description:
Attacks of severe, strictly unilateral pain which is orbital, supraorbital, temporal or in any combination of these sites, lasting 15–180 minutes and occurring from once every other day to eight times a day. The pain is associated with ipsilateral conjunctival injection, lacrimation, nasal congestion, rhinorrhoea, forehead and facial sweating, miosis, ptosis and/or eyelid oedema, and/or with restlessness or agitation.
Diagnostic criteria:
A. At least five attacks fulfilling criteria B–D
B. Severe or very severe unilateral orbital, supraorbital and/or temporal pain lasting 15–180 minutes (when untreated)
C. Either or both of the following:
   1. at least one of the following symptoms or signs, ipsilateral to the headache:
      a) conjunctival injection and/or lacrimation

b) nasal congestion and/or rhinorrhoea
c) eyelid oedema
d) forehead and facial sweating
e) forehead and facial flushing
f) sensation of fullness in the ear
g) miosis and/or ptosis

2. a sense of restlessness or agitation

D. Attacks have a frequency between one every other day and eight per day for more than half of the time when the disorder is active
E. Not better accounted for by another ICHD-3 diagnosis.

3.1.1 Episodic cluster headache
Description:
Cluster headache attacks occurring in periods lasting from 7 days to 1 year, separated by pain-free periods lasting at least 1 month.
Diagnostic criteria:

A. Attacks fulfilling criteria for 3.1 Cluster headache and occurring in bouts (cluster periods)
B. At least two cluster periods lasting from 7 days to 1 year (when untreated) and separated by pain-free remission periods of ≥1 month.

3.1.2 Chronic cluster headache
Description:
Cluster headache attacks occurring for more than 1 year without remission, or with remission periods lasting less than 1 month.
Diagnostic criteria:

A. Attacks fulfilling criteria for 3.1 Cluster headache, and criterion B below
B. Occurring without a remission period, or with remissions lasting <1 month, for at least 1 year.

Appendix B

Methods

I collected the data for this book between 2001 and 2012 using a multisited ethnographic approach. I followed the "idea" of migraine through different sites of cultural representation and knowledge production. My inquiry began with the production of medical knowledge, which involved ethnographic observation at professional headache conferences, interviews with twenty-five experts in the field, analyses of primary historical texts, and targeted literature reviews in contemporary headache medicine. Nearly from the outset, it was clear that medical knowledge could not be separated from the pharmaceutical industry, since these private interests provide treatments, research dollars, and education for doctors, as well as awareness campaigns and advertisements for the public. I soon realized that advocates were also important stakeholders, engaging on every front to increase recognition of headache disorders. Finally, to better understand the cultural logic of migraine, I collected data from cartoons, movies, television, advertisements, common jokes and metaphors, self-help books, and novels. This multisited approach allowed me to examine how medical knowledge, pharmaceutical interests, patient-driven efforts, and cultural representations co-construct how we understand headache disorders.

I included a comparative analysis between migraine and cluster headache to make the gender dynamics embedded in migraine more visible. Cluster headache is a potent foil for migraine. Although cluster headache is undoubtedly a more intense and severe disorder than migraine, the two diagnoses share much in common: their diagnostic criteria and treatment protocols overlap; both are treated by the same specialists; and people with migraine and cluster headache share similar frustrations with pain, suffering, and lack of legitimacy. But migraine and cluster headache are thought to affect different kinds of people. While migraine is often referred to as a "women's disease" (it affects women two to three times more often than it does men), cluster headache is commonly understood to be a "men's disease" (cluster headaches affect men two-and-a-half times as often as women.) Comparing medical, lay, and popular understandings of migraine and cluster headache clarified just how influential gender discourse is in the making of medical knowledge and practice.

Ethnography and Interviews

I began data collection via participant observation at various conferences where members of the headache community gathered to communicate research findings, educate health care providers, and network with each other and with the pharmaceutical industry. In total, I attended ten professional headache conferences, where headache researchers communicated their latest findings, including the 2001, 2003, 2005, and 2009 International Headache Congress, held in New York, Rome, Kyoto, and Philadelphia, respectively; the 2002, 2003, and 2005 American Headache Society (AHS) annual meetings, held in Seattle, Chicago, and Philadelphia; the 2007 AHS annual winter meeting in Scottsdale, Arizona; the 2005 New York Headache Foundation meeting in New York, in which education, rather than scientific communication, was the focus; and the 2003 Cluster Club meeting, held in Rome and meant for scholars and advocates with a specific interest in cluster headache.

Professional headache conferences are usually held in large hotels equipped with massive ballrooms. Invariably, organizers divided these spaces into two separate worlds. Nearly all medical presentations took place in a single ballroom where researchers made back-to-back PowerPoint presentations all day long. The talks were formal, usually involving a panel of speakers at a dais. Audience members never interrupted these talks, waiting instead to ask their questions at the end of the panel. Meanwhile, in a nearby ballroom, pharmaceutical companies and advocacy organizations arranged elaborate displays where representatives answered questions, distributed information, and offered logo-emblazoned gifts to passersby. Sometimes this space was also used for the display of research posters—studies that were of interest to attendees, but which were not given time on the schedule. Coffee and other refreshments were typically located in this room, making it the obvious place for participants to relax, catch up, and network.

At these conferences, I attended talks, viewed research posters, participated in pharmaceutical-sponsored events, and chatted with participants and organizers. I was a bit out of place at these meetings, both as a young woman (most participants were older white men) and as a nonmedical professional. I eventually learned to introduce myself as "something of an anthropologist studying the primitive tribe of headache specialists." This usually made people laugh, putting them at ease. I had countless conversations with participants, engaging researchers and doctors in casual conversation about their work. I used these conversations to ask a variety of questions, including participants' basic beliefs about the cause of headache disorders, how they felt about the direction that headache research is taking, and how they felt about their patients. Their concerns about courtesy stigma and legitimacy emerged spontaneously and often. I also used these conferences as a way to network with and talk to the most prestigious headache specialists. I eventually interviewed twenty-five of the most prominent researchers in American headache medicine. At the time of these interviews, eight of these researchers had already served as president of the AHS, which is the premier scientific organization in the United States dedicated to the study of headache. Almost every other participant was active in another capacity with the AHS, usually as a board member. Four were slated to become president of the organization in the near future. All of these headache specialists had published prolifically in headache medicine, lectured nationally on the subject, served as principal investigators in large-scale research projects on headache disorders, and collaborated with the pharmaceutical industry on major research and educational initiatives. I promised all of these researchers confidentiality. Notably, only three of these twenty-five headache specialists were women. This gender ratio reflects the male dominance of the AHS leadership. For example, of the 2004 AHS Board of Directors, only three of seventeen board members were women, and this included the executive director of AHS, who is a staff member paid to manage the organization. In 2012, Elizabeth Loder became the first woman to serve as president of the organization.

Over the years, I developed important relationships with several headache specialists. Many sought out my expertise in advocacy, policy, and sociology, eventually asked me to provide feedback on manuscripts, congressional testimony, and research proposals. I agreed to submit a chapter to a migraine textbook and to join the AHS's ad hoc committee on "framing migraine," which was charged with developing better ways of communicating migraine to policy makers, employers, and the public. These relationships resulted in informal opportunities for me to learn more about headache medicine. I was able to test my emerging ideas about the development of headache medicine over e-mails, phone calls, dinner parties, texts, and, twice, during journeys to Washington, DC. These conversations revealed a great deal of important background information about the politics and funding of headache medicine.

Medical Literature

I learned a great deal about the social construction of migraine and cluster headache through targeted readings of peer-reviewed journals, medical textbooks, and self-help books written about headache disorders. I read extensively on etiology, epidemiology, and treatments and assiduously followed research published in the two most prominent headache journals, the AHS's journal *Headache* and the International Headache Society's journal *Cephalalgia.* My reading focused on two headache disorders—migraine and cluster headache. My analysis largely excluded other types of headache disorders, for example, tension-type headache, pediatric headache, and chronic daily headache. I also focused my attention on mainstream medicine, excluding alternative approaches to pain control.

In order to situate this reading historically and culturally, I traced the development of migraine and cluster headache medicine as far back as the eighteenth century. Most of this work was completed at the University of Pennsylvania's Biomedical Library. In addition, I spent many additional months doing research in the College of Physicians of Philadelphia Library, the Wellcome Library in London, and New York Weill Cornell Medical Center Archives, where Harold G. Wolff's papers are stored.

Pharmaceutical Advertising

Early on in my research, I realized that the two worlds of headache medicine—medical research and the pharmaceutical industry—were tightly interwoven. Moreover, it was immediately clear to me that these two worlds treated gender in very different ways. At conferences, researchers studiously avoided gratuitous mentions of gender, preferring to illustrate their PowerPoint slides with brains rather than women. At the same time—and in the next room—the pharmaceutical industry pasted their booths, pamphlets, and banners with larger-than-life images of women. I directed my ethnographic efforts toward understanding how these two worlds intersected.

I began by spending hours exploring the pharmaceutical booths. This was always an entertaining part of my fieldwork; booths were often organized as a fairground, each offering passersby games, prizes, amusements, and novelties. Armed with free coffee courtesy of the conference, I would stop and see what was on offer, engaging with materials as though I were a physician. Usually, the booths presented some small select bit of information about a migraine drug. Visitors might then be told that they could have a trinket if they took a short quiz. At other booths, pharmaceutical representatives distributed logo-emblazoned gifts without insisting that any information change hands. I received watches, flash disks, candy, a self-stirring mug, and multiple pieces of "migraine art" to hang in my office. Occasionally, booths offered a "migraine experience," typically a movie or video that attempted to simulate migraine. Some booths—particularly those of companies that made triptans—were extravagant. But many booths consisted of little more than a table with some pamphlets. I stopped at each and every one, collecting pamphlets, gifts, and other cultural objects and asking representatives for more information about their products. In addition, I interviewed two marketing executives who worked at major pharmaceutical companies, both of whom managed marketing for blockbuster migraine medications. Their interviews provided exceedingly helpful background information.

I also attended events that the pharmaceutical industry sponsored beyond the fairground. For example, each conference featured several pharmaceutical-sponsored Continuing Medical Education (CME) events. These panels were funded by unrestricted grants, which purportedly meant that the funder had no say over content. But more often than not, the CME panel would address an issue that had direct relevance to the funding sponsor. For example, an Ortho-McNeil CME event might address the relationship between obesity and migraine. (Ortho-McNeil manufactures topiramate, a Food and Drug Agency–approved preventive medication for migraine that happens to cause weight loss in a subset of patients.) In the evenings, I attended several glamorous events sponsored by these same companies. In New York, I went to an industry-sponsored reception at the Academy of Natural Sciences. In Seattle, I attended a similar reception in the Space Needle. In Italy, I went to an event in Villa Borghese, the gorgeous central park of Rome, where I was entertained by opera singers, clowns on stilts, and a scrumptious three-course meal.

Over time, industry participation in conferences became less extravagant. Ethical concerns about gift giving put the kibosh on the knickknacks that conference participants had gotten used to. And then, as patents on migraine drugs ran out, companies reduced or even eliminated their presence at headache conferences. The fairground became smaller and notably less festive. I heard many grumbles from researchers and conference goers. Companies had, in the past, paid high fees to rent space at conferences, and their funding for CMEs accounted for much of the revenue generated by professional organizations. More than that, though, researchers worried that without migraine drugs on patent, pharmaceutical companies would stop funding their work. These encounters with the pharmaceutical industry revealed the close relationship between industry and headache researchers.

Nevertheless, pharmaceutical companies remain a powerful force (and perhaps the only force) in advertising migraine. To get a sense of what the pharmaceutical industry was saying about migraine, I collected and analyzed advertisements from a wide range of sources. These advertisements provided me with a broad sense of the narratives that companies were using to market their wares, but I also wanted to describe how companies portrayed the average person with migraine. To that end, I conducted a content analysis of images used in a discrete sample of pharmaceutical advertisements. The sample was collected in November 2003—a time when the industry was pouring money into direct-to-consumer advertising for migraine medication. I collected advertisements from a cross section of pharmaceutical websites that market headache medicine—each of which was owned by a company that rented booths at professional headache conferences. I limited my sample to advertising that specifically addressed migraine. I then pared these advertisements down to images from these sites, paying special attention to those that represented the migraine patient and health care workers. I kept all images of people, including both photographs of real people and illustrations or animated representations of people. I discarded all images of objects, such as medication or schematics demonstrating how a medication works. In addition, multiple readings of each website contributed important context for this analysis.

In total, eighty-six images were analyzed. Several images depicted more than one person. The social characteristics of the people depicted were classified according to gender and number (male, alone; female, alone; multiple females; multiple males; mixed), race (white, black, Asian; other, unclear), setting (work—white collar, work—pink collar, work—blue collar, casual, family, clinic, romantic), pain status (pain, nonpain, metaphor for pain, mixed narrative, not applicable), and status (patient, health care provider, expert, other). The location (home page or not) and size (small, medium, or large) of images were also coded. I coded all images alongside a trained independent coder. Inter-coder agreement, calculated using a Kappa statistic, was 89.6 percent (p=.019). I settled all disagreements.

This combination of ethnographic observation and content analysis provided a deep understanding of the role that the pharmaceutical industry plays in constructing the migraine patient.

Online Migraine Communities and Headache Advocacy

Over the years, I followed the activities of headache advocates with great interest. I began by attending the 2003 meeting of the World Headache Alliance (WHA), an umbrella organization for headache advocacy organizations around the world. Advocates from as far as Australia had come to learn more about how they could raise awareness about headache disorders. At that meeting, a headache specialist named Timothy Steiner announced the formation of a new charity called Lifting the Burden, which in collaboration with the World Health Organization sought to measure and raise awareness about the global prevalence of and disability caused by headache disorders. Their efforts have led to a Global Campaign Against Headache.

I soon focused my attention closer to home, attending the 2009, 2010, 2011, and 2012 "Headache on the Hill," sponsored by the American Headache Disorders Alliance (AHDA). The AHDA organizes an annual event in which advocates and patients meet in Washington, DC, to lobby for increased resources to research headache disorders.

I wanted, however, to capture the advocacy efforts of people who had migraine, rather than the efforts of their physicians. I found these grassroots activities on the Internet, which had become an increasingly exciting place for migraine advocacy from 2004 onward. I began by conducting formal interviews with fourteen headache advocates, some of whom run formal organizations (recognized as such by tax status), but most of whom acted alone, either as bloggers or as authors. None of these advocates were promised confidentiality, since they are so accustomed to putting their name to their activities. As such, I use their real name when discussing their comments in the text.

These interviews were helpful, but I learned the most about the collective actions of people with migraine and cluster headache by hanging out online. Advocates maintain online forums where people with migraine and cluster headache can seek help for their symptoms. Bloggers post about their personal experience and readers post comments and questions. Facebook support groups offer spaces where people can vent about migraine and cluster headache. In order to capture these conversations systematically, I collected data from eight headache organizations' websites, including the National Headache Foundation, the American Council for Headache Education, MAGNUM: Migraine Awareness Group: A National Understanding for Migraineurs, the Alliance for Headache Disorders Advocacy, the Migraine Research Foundation, Miles for Migraine, clusterheadaches.com, and Cluster Busters. In April 2012, I downloaded the entirety of twenty-one blogs (ten of which were authored by Teri Robert), including *The Journey of a Migraineur* (http://aloofelf.blogspot.com/), *Somebody Heal Me* (http://somebodyhealme.dianalee.net/), *Fly with Hope* (http://www.flywithhope.com/), *Migraine-ista* (http://migraine-ista.blogspot.com/), *Doc's Cluster Headache Journal* (http://cluster-headache.blogspot.com/), *A Cluster Head's Life* (http://versilleus.blogspot.com/), *The Daily Headache* (www.thedailyheadache.com), *Migraine Truth* (http://migrainetruth.wordpress.com/), *Free My Brain* (http://freemybrain.com/), *Cluster Kate* (http://clusterkate.blogspot.com/), and *That M Word* (http://thatmword.com/). I also wanted to capture ongoing conversations between people with headache disorders, so I downloaded four months of forum conversations on a migraine website and six months of forum conversations on a cluster headache website (time frames were chosen at random).

Analysis

Over the years, I collected tens of thousands of pages of data. That which I could digitize, I imported into a qualitative software program called NVivo. The rest, I sorted into extensive paper files. I followed the guidelines set forth in grounded theory, creating increasingly nuanced themes to help me read through and analyze this data. In the end, I went through many iterations of writing and data analysis before I was satisfied that my argument matched my data.

I also sent some of my chapters to my subjects for review. Two headache specialists read chapter 1 on the history of headache medicine; one of these specialists also read chapter 2, which covered my ethnography of contemporary headache specialists. Two completely different headache specialists read early versions of chapter 4 on migraine advertising and one of these read chapter 5 on cluster headache. One headache advocate read selections of chapter 3. I received overwhelmingly positive feedback from each reader, and most encouraged me to word my arguments in stronger terms. Of course, all errors in the text are mine. I welcome further feedback as this book moves out into the wider world.

Notes

Preface

1. It is quite common for people who have invisible stigmatized conditions to control who knows what about their disorders. Schneider and Conrad referred to this practice as "preventive telling," "In the Closet with Illness."

2. Scher et al., "Prevalence of Frequent Headache in a Population Sample."

3. The experience of receiving random bits of well-meaning, but ill-received advice is so prevalent among those with chronic illness that it has inspired a line of T-shirts and mugs with the tagline "My disabling chronic illness is more real than your imaginary medical expertise."

4. Segal, *Health and the Rhetoric of Medicine*, 40.

5. Greenhalgh, *Under the Medical Gaze*; Ware, "Suffering and the Social Construction of Illness; Werner and Malterud, "It Is Hard Work Behaving as a Credible Patient."

6. Werner and Malterud, "It Is Hard Work Behaving as a Credible Patient," 1409.

7. Moss-Coane, "Radio Times."

8. Mills, *Sociological Imagination*.

9. This approach is informed by standpoint theory. Standpoint theory highlights the position of the researcher and legitimates a more personal social science—one that is produced through an iterative process between data collection, analysis, and self-reflexivity. Standpoint theory has important weaknesses, the most important of which is its tendency to reduce experience to particular identities. Just as not all women are the same, not all people with migraine share the same experiences. Standpoint theory can, however, be useful in its ability to reveal the subjectivities of so-called objective science. See Haraway, "Situated Knowledges"; Harding, "Women's Standpoints on Nature"; Smith, *Conceptual Practices of Power*; Sprague and Zimmerman, "Overcoming Dualisms."

10. Jackson, "'I Am a Fieldnote.'"

11. Evans, Lipton, and Silberstein, "Prevalence of Migraine in Neurologists."

12. Galison and Daston, *Objectivity*.

13. Hustvedt, *Shaking Woman or a History of My Nerves*, 6.

Introduction

1. Burwell, "Pippen Sheds His Wimpy Image."

2. Collins, "Head First."

3. Lichtenstein, "Migraine."

4. Morris, *Culture of Pain*.

5. Osterweis, Kleinman, and Mechanic, *Pain and Disability*.

6. Lipton et al., "Migraine Prevalence, Disease Burden, and the Need for Preventive Therapy."

7. Abu-Arefeh and Russell, "Prevalence of Headache and Migraine in Schoolchildren."

8. Lemos et al., "Assessing Risk Factors for Migraine."

9. Lipton et al. "Prevalence and Burden of Migraine in the United States"; Stewart et al., "Population Variation in Migraine Prevalence"; Silberstein et al., "Probable Migraine in the United States."

10. Lipton et al., "Prevalence and Burden of Migraine in the United States"; Stewart et al., "Population Variation in Migraine Prevalence."

11. Lipton et al., "Migraine Prevalence, Disease Burden, and the Need for Preventive Therapy."

12. Natoli et al., "Global Prevalence of Chronic Migraine."

13. Hirtz et al., "How Common Are the 'Common' Neurologic Disorders?"

14. The American Migraine Study II found that less than 10 percent of those with migraine say that they are able to work or function normally during their attacks. Over half report that their migraines cause severe impairment in activities and require bed rest. Lipton et al., "Prevalence and Burden of Migraine in the United States."

15. Ruiz de Velasco et al., "Quality of Life in Migraine Patients," 894.

16. Ibid., 895.

17. McNell, "Cindy McCain's Secret Struggle with Migraine."

18. Didion, "In Bed." There is nonetheless some (ambiguous) evidence that migraine may be fatal. All forms of migraine slightly increase one's risk of stroke, which can lead to death. A rare form of migraine, basilar artery migraine, increases risk of stroke more significantly. Some advocates argue that migraine ought to be considered fatal because it increases rates of suicide and, indeed, research has demonstrated a link between suicide and migraine pain. See Breslau et al., "Migraine Headaches and Suicide Attempt."

19. Brandes, "Migraine Cycle."

20. Tweedy, "Shaking It Off."

21. Young et al., "Stigma of Migraine."

22. Talcott Parsons's discussion of the sick role argued that sick people had to abide by a set of norms and obligations, including the duty to recognize that their conditions were undesirable and to seek help from a technologically competent healer. These behaviors were cast as moral duties, set forth in order to legitimate illness, which would otherwise be considered a deviant status. Many have noted the limited usefulness of Parsons's sick role in understanding chronic illness. It's a structuralist approach that does not account for historical changes in who is considered sick. It also can't explain chronic illness since people with chronic conditions often fail to get better no matter what kind of help they seek. However, the sick role does highlight the ways in which acquiring legitimacy for sickness is a fundamentally *social* process, produced and negotiated through social interaction with a variety of actors, and which elicits questions about the moral character of the sick person. Parsons, "Social Structure and Dynamic Process."

23. Cooley called this phenomenon "the looking glass self":

> In a very large and interesting class of cases the social reference takes the form of a somewhat definite imagination of how one's self—that is any idea he appropriates—appears in a particular mind, and the kind of self-feeling one has is determined by the attitude toward this attributed to that other mind. A social self of this sort might be called the reflected or looking glass self: "Each to each a looking-glass Reflects the other that doth pass." As we see our face, figure, and dress in the glass, and are interested in them because they are ours, and pleased or otherwise with them according as they do or do not answer to what we should like them to be; so in imagination we perceive in another's mind some thought of our appearance, manners, aims, deeds, character, friends, and so on, and are variously affected by it. (*Human Nature and the Social Order*, 151–52)

24. Kreist, "Engendering Pain."

25. In her study of people with chronic fatigue, Norma Ware argues that the delegitimation of this disorder causes more suffering than the actual disorder itself. Ware, "Suffering and the Social Construction of Illness."

26. Lipton et al., "Migraine Practice Patterns among Neurologists," 1927.

27. "Headache Disorders."

28. Hawkins, Wang, and Rupnow, "Direct Cost Burden among Insured US Employees with Migraine"; Stewart et al., "Lost Productive Time and Cost Due to Common Pain in the US Workforce."

29. "Estimates of Funding for Various Research, Condition, and Disease Categories (RCDC)."

30. The WHO developed DALYs as a metric for comparing the relative burden of diseases. DALYs use time as a metric that includes both years of life lost due to premature death (YLL) and years "lost" due to disability (YLD). Researchers calculated that, on average, people with migraine lost twelve days per year. Schwendt and Shapiro, "Funding of Research on Headache Disorders by the National Institutes of Health."

31. NIH funding per DALY for headache versus other chronic disorders. According to Schwendt and Shapiro, who designed this table, "NIH-funded migraine research received just $29 per DALY attributed to migraine in the United States in 2007. Annual NIH funding per DALY for the ten comparator disorders ranges from $232 to $1,421, with a mean of $734.50. Equivalent annual headache funding would range from $103.5 million to $663.8 million." "Funding of Research on Headache Disorders by the National Institutes of Health," 167.

32. Barker, *Fibromyalgia Story*; Brown, *Toxic Exposures*; Kroll-Smith, Brown, and Gunter, *Illness and the Environment*.

33. Silverman, *Understanding Autism*; Brown, *Toxic Exposures*.

34. Aronowitz, *Making Sense of Illness*; Brown, "Naming and Framing"; Freidson, *Profession of Medicine*; Rosenberg and Golden, "Framing Disease."

35. Rosenberg, "Contested Boundaries."

36. Conrad, *The Medicalization of Society*.

37. Troyer, "Legitimacy."

38. Aronowitz, *Making Sense of Illness*; Rosenberg and Golden, *Framing Disease*.

39. Aronowitz, *Making Sense of Illness*.

40. Conrad, "Discovery of Hyperkinesis." To read more about the relationship between drug development and disease creation, see also Greene, *Prescribing by the Numbers*.

41. Dumit, *Picturing Personhood*; Joyce, *Magnetic Appeal*.

42. Aronowitz, *Making Sense of Illness*.

43. Barker, *Fibromyalgia Story*; Rosenberg, "Tyranny of Diagnosis"; Jutel, *Putting a Name to It*; Brown, "Naming and Framing."

44. Barker, *Fibromyalgia Story*.

45. Goffman, *Stigma*.

46. Dumit, "Illnesses You Have to Fight to Get."

47. Hoffman and Tarzian, "The Girl Who Cried Pain."

48. Loder and Beluk, "Influence of Gender on Evaluation and Treatment of Migraine."

49. Crook and Tunks, "Women with Pain"; Hoffman and Tarzian, "The Girl Who Cried Pain."

50. Wailoo, *Dying in the City of the Blues*.

51. Best, "Disease Politics and Medical Research Funding."

52. Martin, *Woman in the Body*; Richardson, "Sexing the X"; Schiebinger, *Mind Has No Sex?*

53. Martin, *Woman in the Body*; Simonds, Rothman, and Norman, *Laboring On*.

54. Martin, *Flexible Bodies*.

55. Blum and Stracuzzi, "Gender in the Prozac Nation"; Metzl, *Prozac on the Couch*.

56. Butler, *Bodies That Matter.*

57. Agonito, *History of Ideas on Woman*; Okin, *Women in Western Political Thought*; Spanier, *Im/Partial Science*; Harding, *Science Question in Feminism*.

58. Scott, "Gender."

59. See appendix B for more details on methodology.

60. Swidler, "Culture in Action."

61. Fifteen other synonyms listed (of nineteen total) ("aggravation," "bore," "bother," "burdensome," "distress," "misery," "nuisance," "onerous," "oppressive," "pest," "problem," "task," "tribulation," "woe," "worry") speak to the low status accorded to headache by reflecting a commonsense understanding that headache is something irritating, but nothing of grave concern.

62. Geertz, "Ideology as a Cultural System," 211.

63. Couch and Bearss, "Relief of Migraine Headache with Sexual Orgasm."

64. Fulbright, "Sexpert Q&A."

Chapter One

1. Grant's story is frequently invoked in articles and books about migraine. See, for example, Kiester, "Doctors Close in on the Mechanisms Behind Headache." General Ulysses S. Grant's account can be found in his diary, *Personal Memoirs of Ulysses S. Grant*, 430–31.

2. The so-called let-down migraine or weekend headache may not be caused by a change in affect. These migraines might be triggered by a behavioral change on the weekends, like sleeping late, rather than actual relaxation. But it is easy to perceive these features of migraine as products of the mind.

3. Didion, "In Bed," 172.

4. Davidoff, *Migraine*.

5. Hustvedt, "Lifting, Lights and Little People."

6. Sacks, "Patterns."

7. Carroll, *Alice in Wonderland*, 6.

8. Sacks, *Migraine*, viii.

9. As mind is increasingly understood to be brain, the mind/body "continuum" has ceased to be so linear.

10. Treichler, *How to Have Theory in an Epidemic*, 43.

11. Headache disorders, many of which sound like modern-day migraine, were known by a variety of terms, including megrim, sick headache, nervous headache, and clavus hystericus.

12. Plato, *Charmides.*

13. Isler, "Galenic Tradition and Migraine," 227.

14. Willis, *London Practice of Physick*, 371.

15. Eadie, "18th Century Understanding of Migraine," 414.

16. Mease, *Causes, Cure, and Prevention of the Sick-Headache*, 43.

17. Rosenberg, "Body and Mind in Nineteenth-Century Medicine," 185–97.

18. Symonds, "Gulstonian Lectures at the Royal College of Physicians," 287.

19. Ibid., 287.

20. Ibid., 395–96.

21. Barker-Benfield, *Culture of Sensibility.*

22. Cheyne, *English Malady*, 46.

23. Ibid., 71.

24. Ibid., 37.

25. Ibid.

26. Barker-Benfield, *Culture of Sensibility.*

27. Mandeville, *Treatise of the Hypochondriack and Hysterick Diseases*, 238–39.

28. Cheyne, *English Malady*, 14.

29. Austen, *Sense and Sensibility.*

30. Symonds, "Gulstonian Lectures at the Royal College of Physicians," 287.

31. Symonds was no doubt influenced by a broader discussion in medicine about a condition called "neuromimesis," in which it was thought that people with weak nervous systems could "catch" a disease by mere suggestion. See Vrettos, *Somatic Fictions.*

32. Koehler, "Brown-Sequard's Comment on Du Bois-Reymond's 'Hemikrania Sympathicotonica.' "

33. Latham, *On Nervous or Sick-Headache*, 17.

34. Ibid., 20.

35. Liveing, *On Megrim, Sick-Headache and Some Allied* Disorders, 337.

36. Pearce, "Edward Liveing's (1832–1919) Theory of Nerve-Storms in Migraine."

37. Especially Sacks, *Migraine.*

38. Latham, *On Nervous or Sick-Headache*, 20.

39. Ibid., 15.

40. Ibid.

41. The metaphorical connection between emotions and the vascular system extend at least back to Hippocratic writings, which suggested that every feeling gov-

erns an organ. "Anger, for example, contracts and good feelings dilate the heart." Ackerknecht, "History of Psychosomatic Medicine," 17.

42. Liveing, *On Megrim, Sick-Headache and Some Allied Disorders*, 26.

43. Ibid., 35.

44. Ibid., 26.

45. Kempner, "Sociologic Perspective in Migraine in Women"; Segal, *Health and the Rhetoric of Medicine*.

46. Symonds, "Gulstonian Lectures at the Royal College of Physicians," 497.

47. Liveing, *On Megrim, Sick-Headache and Some Allied Disorders*, 23.

48. Ross, *Treatise on the Diseases of the Nervous System*, 544.

49. Hamilton, *Modern Treatment of Headaches*, 105.

50. Ibid., 106.

51. Although Freud (another of many migraine sufferers) wrote that migraine was an actual neurosis and had no subconscious psychic meaning, his work inspired several psychodynamic theories of migraine. Franz Alexander, in *Psychosomatic Medicine*, argued that migraine was a regressive reaction, marked by helplessness. Others wrote that migraine represented an encapsulative event, in which the stressors of the month may be dealt with in one migraine. In other words, migraine served as a reset button to relieve a stressed nervous system. Even Sacks with his neurological orientation suggests something similar in the preface of his 1970 edition of *Migraine*: "migraine as a *structure* whose forms were implicit in the repertoire of the nervous system and as a *strategy* which might be employed to any emotional or indeed biological end," xviii.

52. McTavish, "Pain and Profits."

53. Ergotamine has been in use since 1880. William Gowers recommended ergotamine for migraine treatment in 1908. However, it did not become popular for migraine treatment until the 1930s, when crystalline preparations were made available. Dihydroergotamine (DHE) is an ergotamine derivative that continues to be used in the abortive treatment of migraine. Gowers, *Borderland of Epilepsy*; Sacks, *Migraine*; Silberstein, "Ergotamine and Dihydroergotamine."

54. Wolff's historical importance has been recognized by the American Headache Society, which named its most prestigious annual award after him. His reference book, *Headache and Other Head Pain*, is in its sixth revised edition. Wolff also published extensively in the psychosomatic literature. See for example, Wolff, *Stress and Disease*; Wolff and Wolf, *Pain*.

55. Goodell, "Thirty Years of Headache Research in the Laboratory of the Late Dr. Harold G. Wolff."

56. Ibid., 161.

57. Wolff, *Headache and Other Head Pain*. A 1966 article in the journal *Headache* begins by describing classic migraine: "At the present day, it is generally held

that migraine is a vascular disorder including vasospastic and vasoparetic events combined with oedema of the vessel wall." Cited in Bruyn and Weenink, "Migraine Accompagnee," 1.

58. Goodell and Wolff, "Influence on Medicine and Neurology of Harold G. Wolff."

59. Wolff, cited in Goodell, "Thirty Years of Headache Research in the Laboratory of the Late Dr. Harold G. Wolff," 159.

60. Goodell, "Thirty Years of Headache Research in the Laboratory of the Late Dr. Harold G. Wolff."

61. Selinsky, "Psychologic Study of the Migrainous Syndrome," 759.

62. This comment appears as a handwritten reminder at the end of Wolff's typed lecture notes to his second-year medical students in 1939. Wolff, *New York Weill Cornell Medical Center Archives*, "Box 15, Folder 2."

63. Wolff, *Headache and Other Head Pain*, 401–2.

64. Foucault, *Discipline and Punish*.

65. Wolff, *Headache and Other Head Pain* dedicates a chapter to characterizations such as these, 399–431.

66. Furnas, "Headaches Are a Luxury," 145.

67. Wolff, *New York Weill Cornell Medical Center Archives*, "Box 16, Folder 10."

68. Goodell, "Thirty Years of Headache Research in the Laboratory of the Late Dr. Harold G. Wolff," 162.

69. Segal, *Health and the Rhetoric of Medicine*.

70. Wolff, *Headache and Other Head Pain*, 415.

71. Ibid., 416.

72. Ibid., 412.

73. Ibid., 414–15.

74. Reilly, *Headache*.

75. Alvarez, "Notes on the History of Migraine."

76. Kunkel, "American Headache Society."

77. Alvarez, "Migrainous Woman and All Her Troubles."

78. Ibid., 3.

79. Ibid., 4–5.

80. Ibid., 6.

81. Ibid., 5.

82. Ibid., 4–5.

83. Ibid., 4.

84. Ad Hoc Committee on Classification of Headache. "Classification of Headache," 127.

85. Garner, Shulman, and Diamond, "Psychiatric Aspects of Headache."

86. Ibid., 2.

87. Ibid.

88. Ibid., 3.

89. Ibid., 9–10.

90. Segal, *Health and the Rhetoric of Medicine.*

91. Hacking, *Social Construction of What?*

92. Didion, "In Bed," 171.

93. Lance, *Mechanism and Management of Headache*; Lance, Anthony, and Hinterberger, "Control of Cranial Arteries by Humoral Mechanisms and Its Relation to the Migraine Syndrome"; Sicuteri, "Prophylactic and Therapeutic Properties of Methyl Lysergic Acid Butanolamide in Migraine."

94. Raskin, "Conclusions," 24.

95. Aronowitz, *Making Sense of Illness.*

96. Lance, *Mechanism and Management of Headache*, 000. He also discusses this in an earlier paper, Lance and Anthony, "Some Clinical Aspects of Migraine."

97. Waters and O'Connor, "Epidemiology of Headache and Migraine in Women."

98. Elithorn, "Migraine," 411.

99. Diamond and Dalessio, *Practicing Physician's Approach to Headache.*

100. Saper and Magee, *Freedom from Headaches*, 82.

101. Ibid.

102. Packard, "Psychiatric Aspects of Headache," 169.

103. South and Sheftell "Communicating with the Patient," 604.

104. Buchholz, *Heal Your Headache*, 43. Physicians have several effective pharmaceutical methods for helping patients cope with withdrawal symptoms.

105. Ibid., 185.

106. Ibid., 184.

107. Ibid.

108. Andreasen, *Broken Brain.*

109. Ibid.; Luhrmann, *Of Two Minds.*

110. Rose, *Politics of Life Itself*, 192.

111. Silberstein and Rothrock, *State of Migraine*, 5.

112. Goadsby, Lipton, and Ferrari, "Migraine—Current Understanding and Treatment." However, recent research indicates that the vascular system plays no role in migraine. See Amin et al., "Magnetic Resonance Angiography of Intracranial and Extracranial Arteries in Patients with Spontaneous Migraine without Aura."

113. Pearce, "Edward Liveing's (1832–1919) Theory of Nerve-Storms in Migraine."

114. It is important to note, however, that so-called antidepressants are not specific to clinically diagnosed cases of depression. Nevertheless, the use of these drugs on migraine may suggest that the two disorders share an underlying biological mechanism

115. Sontag, *Illness as Metaphor and AIDS and Its Metaphors.*

116. Lakoff and Johnson, *Metaphors We Live By.*

Chapter Two

1. Science studies scholars might call this a "credibility crisis." The literature on credibility in science has been useful in my analysis, helping me understand how scientists go about using particular kinds of evidence and rhetoric to establish their credibility. However, I talk about legitimacy in headache medicine because this is the term that headache specialists use to describe their own predicament. It is also a useful term because it emphasizes the link between the credibility of headache medicine as a profession and the ontology of migraine. Latour and Woolgar, *Laboratory Life*; Fujimura, *Crafting Science*; Epstein, *Impure Science*; Porter, *Trust in Numbers*.

2. Liveing, *On Megrim, Sick-Headache and Some Allied Disorders*, iv.

3. Leyton, *Migraine and Periodic Headache*, 106.

4. Rothrock, "In This Issue," 669.

5. Lipton et al., "Migraine Practice Patterns among Neurologists," 1929.

6. Shapiro and Goadsby, "Long Drought." In comparison, the American Epilepsy Society boasts 1,940 US members, most of whom are neurologists. Kathy Hucks, membership coordinator of the American Epilepsy Society, e-mail to author, July 20, 2012.

7. Sheftell and Tepper, "New Paradigms in the Recognition and Acute Treatment of Migraine," 58.

8. Finkel, "American Academic Headache Specialists in Neurology"; "Atlas of Headache Disorders and Resources in the World 2011."

9. Kommineni and Finkel, "Teaching Headache in America."

10. Drexler, *New Approaches to Neurological Pain*, 3.

11. Of course, almost no headache specialists have "special training" since fellowships in headache medicine were only instituted in 2006. Finkel, "Legitimization of Headache Medicine."

12. Kommineni and Finkel, "Teaching Headache in America."

13. Appenzeller, "No Appointment Needed," 133.

14. Rosen and Mauser, "So Many Migraines, So Few Specialists."

15. "Money losing" does not mean that these headache specialists aren't earning six-figure salaries, although many respondents complained that they earned less than neurologists in other specialties.

16. Baszanger, *Inventing Pain Medicine,* 111.

17. Barker, *Fibromyalgia Story*.

18. Baszenger, *Inventing Pain Medicine*, 112.

19. This quote was taken from Silberstein, Lipton, and Goadsby, *Headache in Clinical Practice*, 5, but I heard and read permutations of it used often, for example, by Sheftell, World Headache Alliance meeting, fieldnotes, September 10, 2003, and L'Europa, *Stop Limiting Migraine Medicine.*

20. Norredam and Album, "Prestige and Its Significance for Medical Specialties and Diseases."

21. Album and Westin, "Do Diseases Have a Prestige Hierarchy?"

22. Bendelow, *Pain and Gender*, found that members of the UK public also stratified by types of pain, with physical pain trumping emotional pain.

23. Goffman, *Stigma*, 30.

24. Finkel, "Legitimization of Headache Medicine," 711.

25. Carr, "Enactments of Expertise."

26. Rosenberg, "Tyranny of Diagnosis," 238.

27. Martin, "Talking Back to Neuro-reductionism."

28. Abbott, *System of Professions.*

29. Robert S. Kunkel, phone call with author, September 1, 2009.

30. Ibid.

31. Kunkel, "American Headache Society," 681.

32. Linda McGillicuddy, e-mail to author, February 1, 2012.

33. Ad Hoc Committee on Classification of Headache, "Classification of Headache."

34. Olesen, "International Classification of Headache Disorders," 691.

35. Cutrer, "Functional Imaging in Primary Headache Disorders," 704.

36. Wessman et al., "Migraine."

37. Ophoff et al., "Familial Hemiplegic Migraine and Episodic Ataxia Type-2 Are Caused by Mutations in the Ca2+ Channel Gene Cacn11a4."

38. de Vries et al., "Molecular Genetics of Migraine."

39. Cady et al., "Treatment of Acute Migraine with Subcutaneous Sumatriptan."

40. Humphrey, "Discovery and Development of Triptans, a Major Therapeutic Breakthrough," 685.

41. Ibid.

42. Ibid.

43. See Weiner et al., "Attributional Analysis of Reactions to Stigmas"; Rush, "Affective Reactions to Multiple Social Stigmas"; Corrigan et al., "Stigmatizing Attributions about Mental Illness."

44. Dumit, *Picturing Personhood*, 166.

45. Moss-Coane, "Radio Times."

46. Phillips, "Migraine as a Woman's Issue—Will Research and New Treatments Help?," 1975.

47. Casting the brain in opposition to femininity might seem strange in light of feminist criticism that has long held that the body is the "prototype of feminine concrete existence." But as Martin points out, neuroreductionism reconfigures the body in masculine terms, making it "universal, unhistorical, unconscious of its own production, and possessed of many of the characteristics of modernist

scientific accounts. . . . The brain has become sovereign and its sovereignty conceals what Geertz argued in 1962: that the human brain is a product of a *relation with culture.*" Martin, "Mind-Body Problems," 576.

48. For a critical review of this research, see Jordan-Young, *Brain Storm.*

49. American Headache Society, accessed March 18, 2004, www.ahs.net.

50. Gieryn, "Boundary-Work and the Demarcation of Science from Non-Science."

51. Phelan, "Geneticization of Deviant Behavior and Consequences for Stigma," 316.

52. Pescosolido et al., " 'A Disease like Any Other'?"

53. Bernstein and McArdle, *Migraine Brain*, 40.

54. "Stink over Perfume at Detroit Workplace."

55. Silberstein and Rothrock, *State of Migraine*, 8.

56. HealthTalk Webcast, "What Causes Migraine Headaches?"

57. Livingstone and Novak, *Breaking the Headache Cycle*, 47.

58. Cady, "Migraines and Emotional Health."

59. Ibid.

60. Ibid.

61. Cheyne, *English Malady.*

Chapter Three

1. I use the real names of migraine advocates and bloggers who post content to the Internet, since they make their work available to the public. However, I anonymize comments from those who contribute to forums or comment on blogs, since they have not positioned themselves as opinion leaders in the community. Although they, too, are posting content that is available to the public, I doubt that any of the users of these forums thought that their comments would be published when they pressed enter. Unfortunately, in an era when identities can be uncovered with a simple Google search, anonymizing has required that I paraphrase their contributions. The inevitable outcome is that their edited comments dilute the power of their experiences and opinions. To compensate, I draw more heavily on interview and blog data to represent similar sentiments that I found on forums.

2. Kleinman, "Pain and Resistance"; Lillrank, "Back Pain and the Resolution of Diagnostic Uncertainty in Illness Narratives"; Morris, *Culture of Pain*; Scarry, *Body in Pain*; Whelan, " 'No One Agrees except for Those of Us Who Have It.' "

3. Cooper, "Myalgic Encephalomyelitis and the Medical Encounter," 202.

4. One might assume that this experience is also racialized and classed, but exactly how it breaks down by race and class is not well understood. For a good overview of how women are often ignored when they complain about pain, see Hoffman and Tarzian, "Girl Who Cried Pain."

5. Barker, "Self-Help Literature and the Making of an Illness Identity."

6. Robert, "Migraine Research Funding—An Important Step."

7. Rabinow, "Artificiality and Enlightenment."

8. Brown et al., "Embodied Health Movements."

9. Prior to these efforts, organizations devoted to helping migraine patients, were led by physicians, not patients. In the United States, the largest and oldest such organization is the National Headache Foundation (NHF). Similarly, physicians run the American Council for Headache Education (ACHE)—a "patient education center." The first and only American patient-run advocacy organization for migraine is MAGNUM (short for Migraine Awareness Group: A National Understanding for Migraineurs). MAGNUM is a small organization that has, in the past, done some lobbying, but which currently has no members.

10. On June 7, 2012, Amazon.com listed Robert's book as the third most popular book in the headache category, after Buchholz's *Heal Your Headache* and a book on acupuncture for headache.

11. I also work for Health Union, LLC, as an occasional blogger for their website Migraine.com.

12. Chris Regal, personal communication with author, April 23, 2012.

13. Teri Robert, personal communication with author, April 20, 2012.

14. Race and ethnicity are difficult to parse from online interactions, but the moderators are overwhelmingly white.

15. One electronic support group formed an organization called the PFO Research Foundation. PFO is short for patent foramen ovale, which is a small opening in the wall of the heart that separates the top two chambers. PFOs are thought to be relatively common in humans and are associated with migraine. I do not include this organization in my analysis, however, because the PFO Research Foundation is organized around this heart defect, rather than around migraine.

16. Evans and Boyte, *Free Spaces*, 17.

17. Somers calls these stories "ontological narratives" in "Narrative Constitution of Identity."

18. Ibid.

19. Frank, *Wounded Storyteller*.

20. Katzenstein, "Discursive Politics and Feminist Activism in the Catholic Church."

21. Robert, "Elvis and LSD?"

22. Schnakenberg, "Migraine Dirty Dozen—Things Not to Say to a Chronic Migraineur."

23. Zanitsch, "Stop the Insanity."

24. Schnakenberg, "Why Does the Emergency Room Treat Me like a Drug Seeker?"

25. Smyres, "Day-to-Day Life of a Chronic Migraineur."

26. Ibid.

27. Smyres, "Requesting Accommodations Eases Burden of Disability."

28. Wahle, "Five Things That Changed My Life."

29. Leeloo, "Migraine and Suicide."

30. Dumit, *Picturing Personhood*, 7.

31. Rose, *Politics of Life Itself.*

32. Petryna describes biological citizenship as state and political recognition of people based on biological characteristics in *Life Exposed*. In contrast, Rose and Novas describe biological citizenship as the way that biotechnology restructures how we understand our selves in "Biological Citizenship." Migraine advocates restructure how they conceive of themselves in order to be recognized politically, socially, and economically.

33. Lee, "Finding the Right Migraine Preventive Medication Is Complicated, Frustrating."

34. Individuals in embodied health movements are also highly reliant on medicine and, therefore, are unlikely to make doctors their enemies, even as they critique dominant epidemiological models of medicine. In migraine, however, there is very little critique of dominant epidemiological models. Bell, *DES Daughters, Embodied Knowledge, and the Transformation of Women's Health Politics in the Late Twentieth Century*; Brown, "Popular Epidemiology and Toxic Waste Contamination."

35. Schnakenberg, "Migraine Milestones."

36. Not all online communities agree about which biomedical knowledge ought to be adopted and which knowledge ought to be rejected. However, this variation can often be attributed to how the communities position themselves vis-à-vis the legitimacy deficit. For example, Teri Robert, who has found success in mainstream headache medicine, has adopted headache specialists' claim that opioid drugs are terrible treatments for migraine and ought never be used, as they often cause migraine to progress into something much worse. However, other communities reject this knowledge, arguing that opioids are sometimes needed and that doctors only withhold these drugs because migraine patients are viewed as addicts. See, for example, Catherine Charrett-Dykes's blog post on this, "Chronic Migraine and Suicide Awareness Day," in which she says, "There are some in the medical field that believe they are doing us a favor by not prescribing narcotics because of fear of addiction. There is a physical component to addiction . . . but there's an even bigger physical component to pain."

37. Bell finds that embodied health movements often embrace medical paradigms, too. *DES Daughters, Embodied Knowledge, and the Transformation of Women's Health Politics in the Late Twentieth Century.*

38. Lipton and Pan, "Is Migraine a Progressive Brain Disease?"

39. de Vries et al., "Molecular Genetics of Migraine."

40. Young et al., "Naming Migraine and Those Who Have It."

41. Schürks et al., "Migraine and Cardiovascular Disease."

42. See Robert, *Living Well with Migraine Disease and Headaches.*

43. Scarry talks about the "kinship between pain and death, both of which are radical and absolute. . . . [There is] an intuitive human recognition that pain is the equivalent in felt-experience of what is unfeelable in death. . . . Physical pain always mimes death." *Body in Pain*, 31.

44. Breslau et al., "Migraine Headaches and Suicide Attempt."

45. Schnakenberg, "Why Is Migraine Capitalized?"

46. Robert, "Understanding Migraine Disease and Migraineurs."

47. Robert, "10 Things I Want to Share about Migraines."

48. Morgan, "Migraine Battle Continues."

49. Ibid.

50. Smyres, "Not Just a Headache."

51. Schnakenberg, "Migraine and the ER—A Follow-Up Interview."

52. Robert, "Understanding Migraine Disease and Migraineurs."

53. Valendy, "Elevator Blog."

54. "Tea for Two or the World Is My Teacup."

55. Robert, "Defeated, Hopeless, Powerless, Useless—Migraine in a Word."

56. Oltman, "It's All In Your Head."

57. Scarry discusses how pain always seems to come outside of oneself; the body becomes "the agent of his agony." The same is true, here, in migraine. *Body in Pain*, 47.

58. Geddis, "Ten Days and Counting."

59. Lee, "Migraineurs."

60. Curtis, "Blogger's Choice."

61. Brown et al., "Embodied Health Movements."

62. Vidal, "Brainhood, Anthropological Figure of Modernity."

63. Lipton et al., "Migraine Diagnosis and Treatment."

64. Bigal et al., "Migraine in Adolescents."

65. Curtis, Pamela, "Blogger's Choice."

Chapter Four

1. Goffman, *Gender Advertisements*; Bordo, *Unbearable Weight.*

2. Prather and Fidell, "Sex Differences in the Content and Style of Medical Advertisements"; Hawkins and Aber, "Content of Advertisements in Medical Journals."

3. Mant and Darroch, "Media Images and Medical Images"; Curry and O'Brien, "Male Heart and the Female Mind."

4. Lupton, "Construction of Patienthood in Medical Advertising."

5. Whittaker, "Re-Framing the Representation of Women in Advertisements for Hormone Replacement Therapy," 81.

6. Greene, *Prescribing by the Numbers*; Conrad and Leiter, "Medicalization, Markets and Consumers"; Barker, "Listening to Lyrica"; Williams, Gabe, and Davis, "Sociology of Pharmaceuticals."

7. Berkrot, "Global Drug Sales to Top $1 Trillion in 2014."

8. Gatyas, "Modest Rise in Real Per Capita Spending."

9. Angell, *Truth about Drug Companies*.

10. Gagnon and Lexchin, "Cost of Pushing Pills."

11. McTavish, *Pain and Profits*.

12. Sahoo, "Lifecycle Management Strategies."

13. Williams, Martin, and Gabe, "Pharmaceuticalisation of Society?"

14. Ibid., 711.

15. In the United Kingdom, one may now buy Imigran over the counter, under limited circumstances. GlaxoSmithKline, "Proposed Merger of GlaxoWellcome and SmithKline Beecham."

16. Ferrari et al., "Oral Triptans (Serotonin 5-HT1B/1D Agonists) in Acute Migraine Treatment."

17. For each IHS and AHS president serving since 2001, I counted the number of conflicts of interests that they self-reported on published articles and Continuing Medical Education programs. These figures are likely underestimates, as the AHS only required its members to state conflict of interests in 2006.

18. Olesen et al., "Funding of Headache Research in Europe."

19. "Estimates of Funding for Various Research, Condition, and Disease Categories (RCDC)."

20. Pines, "History and Perspective on Direct-to-Consumer Promotion."

21. Ibid.

22. Frank et al., "Trends in Direct-to-Consumer Advertising of Prescription Drugs."

23. Liu and Ducette, "Does Direct-to-Consumer Advertising Affect Patient's Choice of Pain Medication?"

24. Krajnak, "Glaxo Wellcome."

25. Angell, *Truth about Drug Companies*.

26. Ibid.; Goodman, "Celebrity Pill Pushers."

27. See Sismondo, "Ghost Management."

28. For a historical perspective on how marketing infuses the research and development of pharmaceuticals, see Greene, *Prescribing by the Numbers*.

29. Gagnon and Lexchin, "Cost of Pushing Pills."

30. A full accounting of these methods is available in the appendix.

31. "Understanding the Root of your Pain," Accessed September 10, 2003, http://www.migrainehelp.com./2.understanding_migraine/2.1.understanding_migraines.html

32. Hawkins and Aber, "Content of Advertisements in Medical Journals"; Lovdahl, Riska, and Riska, "Gender Display in Scandinavian and American Ad-

vertising for Antidepressants"; Lupton, "Construction of Patienthood in Medical Advertising"; Metzl, *Prozac on the Couch*; Whittaker, "Re-framing the Representation of Women in Advertisements for Hormone Replacement Therapy."

33. Goffman, *Gender Advertisements.*

34. "Toughing It Out: Wondering What Others Think," Accessed September 15, 2003, http://migrainerelief.com/harrispoll_04.html.

35. "Who Suffers: An Office Snapshot . . . ," Accessed September 15, 2003, http://migrainerelief.com/basics_definitions.html#who_suffers.

36. Lipton et al., "Prevalence and Burden of Migraine in the United States"; Silberstein et al., "Probable Migraine in the United States."

37. Riska, "Gender and Medicalization and Biomedicalization Theories"; Bell and Figert, "Gender and the Medicalization of Healthcare."

38. Lakoff and Johnson, *Metaphors We Live By*; Geertz, "Ideology as a Cultural System."

39. Muilenburg, "National Headache Foundation, Healthy Women and Allergan Announce First Winner of National 'Rewrite Your Day' Educational Campaign and Contest for People Living with Chronic Migraine."

40. "Pfizer Gives Its New Relpax Drug the Spa Treatment."

41. Ibid.

42. www.relpax.com.

43. Riska, *Masculinity and Men's Health.*

44. Martin, "Pharmaceutical Person."

45. Binder, "Constructing Racial Rhetoric"; Gamson and Modigliani, "Media Discourse and Public Opinion on Nuclear Power"; Schudson, "How Culture Works."

46. Martin, "Pharmaceutical Person."

47. Metzl, *Prozac on the Couch.*

48. Ibid.

49. National Center for Health Statistics, "Current Estimates from the National Health Interview Survey, 1996."

50. Insurance companies limited most patients to nine tablets per month, which became a problem for millions of people whose doctors prescribed considerably more than this.

51. Barker, "Listening to Lyrica."

Chapter Five

1. Steinem, "If Men Could Menstruate."

2. Dodick et al., "Cluster Headache."

3. Bahra, May, and Goadsby, "Cluster Headache."

4. Dodick et al., "Cluster Headache," 788.

5. Saper and Magee, *Freedom from Headaches*, 113.

6. Classification Committee of the International Headache Society, "International Classification of Headache Disorders, 3rd Edition."

7. D'Alessandro et al., "Cluster Headache in the Republic of San Marino"; Ekbom et al., "Age at Onset and Sex Ratio in Cluster Headache"; Kudrow, *Cluster Headache*; Noonan, Kathman, and White, "Prevalence Estimates for MS in the United States and Evidence of an Increasing Trend for Women."

8. Rapoport, Sheftell, and Tepper, *Conquering Headache*, 13.

9. Sjaastad, *Cluster Headache Syndrome*, 30.

10. Graham, "Cluster Headache," 181.

11. Saper, *Headache Disorders*, 104.

12. Graham, "Cluster Headache"; Manzoni, "Gender Ratio of Cluster Headache over the Years."

13. Sjoberg et al., "Case Study Approach in Social Research."

14. Saper and Magee, *Freedom from Headaches*, 113.

15. Kudrow, *Cluster Headache*, 26.

16. Bahra, May, and Goadsby, "Cluster Headache," 358.

17. Anonymous, clusterheadaches.com.

18. Goadsby, "Pathophysiology of Cluster Headache," 251.

19. Many women with migraine also say that their pain is worse than childbirth. This strikes me as an odd comparison for a number of reasons. First, women's experience of childbirth is highly variable and depends on a number of factors including the baby's position, size of pelvis, use of painkillers, length of labor, and so forth. Second, pain is rarely experienced without emotion. I had a chance to reflect on this during the birth of my son. The two pains (that of migraine and that of child birth) struck me at the time and then again, on reflection, as utterly different experiences, rendering the comparison nonsense. I look back on my labor with considerable nostalgia. Yes, there was intense pain and, yes, it went on for three long days. But it was also exciting, frightening, nerve-wracking, and utterly transformative. In contrast, I remain somewhat traumatized by the twice-weekly migraines that left me in bed for much of my first trimester. And yet, I cannot say that these migraines were more painful than childbirth—but they did cause much more suffering.

20. Saper, "Nonheadache Disorders and Characteristics of Cluster Headache Patients."

21. Koehler, "Prevalence of Headache in Tulp's Observationes Medicae (1641) with a Description of Cluster Headache."

22. Isler, "Episodic Cluster Headache from a Textbook of 1745."

23. See Bing, *Lehrbuch der Nervenkrankheiten*; Boes et al., "Wilfred Harris' Early Description of Cluster Headache."

24. Kunkle, Wilhoit, and Hamrick, "Recurrent Brief Headache in Cluster Pattern."

25. Many people with cluster headache say that their attacks are not predictable and contest this "alarm clock" moniker.

26. Wolff, *Headache and Other Head Pain*, 514.

27. Friedman, "Cluster Headaches," 656.

28. In Nieman and Hurwitz's study, only seven of forty-seven cluster patients regarded worry, overwork, or stress as a provocative trigger. "Ocular Sympathetic Palsy in Perodic Migrainous Neuralgia." F. Schiller found that only a small portion of his fifty-two cluster patients suffered from anxiety or had compulsive, phobic characteristics. "Prophylactic and Other Treatment for 'Histaminic Cluster' or Limited Variant of Migraine."

29. Graham published this research in 1972 in an article titled "Cluster Headache."

30. Ibid., 182.

31. Ibid.

32. Ibid., 178.

33. Ibid., 181.

34. Ibid., 184.

35. Kudrow, "Physical and Personality Characteristics in Cluster Headache."

36. Ibid, 198.

37. Kudrow, *Cluster Headache*, 43.

38. Kudrow and Sutkus, "MMPI Pattern Specificity in Primary Headache Disorders."

39. Andrasik, Blanchard, and Arena, "Cross-Validation of the Kudrow-Sutkus MMPI Classification System for Diagnosing Headache Type"; Blanchard and Andrasik, *Management of Chronic Headaches*; Cuypers, Alternkirch, and Bunge, "Personality Profiles in Cluster Headache and Migraine"; Pfaffenrath et al., "MMPI Personality Profiles in Patients with Primary Headache Syndromes."

40. Harrison, "Psychological Testing in Headache"; Merskey et al., "Psychological Normality and Abnormality in Persistent Headache Patients"; Robinson et al., "Relationship between MMPI Cluster Membership and Diagnostic Category in Headache Patients."

41. Bertolotti et al., "Psychological and Emotional Aspects and Pain"; Harrison, "Warning"; Robinson et al., "Relationship between MMPI Cluster Membership and Diagnostic Category in Headache Patients."

42. Saper, "Nonheadache Disorders and Characteristics of Cluster Headache Patients."

43. Italian Cooperative Study Group on the Epidemiology of Cluster Headache, "Case-control Study on the Epidemiology of Cluster Headache II."

44. Ekbom et al., "Age at Onset and Sex Ratio in Cluster Headache"; Friedman, "Cluster Headaches"; Kudrow, *Cluster Headache*; Lovshin, "Clinical Caprices of Histaminic Cephalgia."

45. Bahra, May, and Goadsby, "Cluster Headache"; Manzoni, "Male Preponderance of Cluster Headache Is Progressively Decreasing over the Years"; Manzoni, "Gender Ratio of Cluster Headache over the Years."

46. Levi et al., "Episodic Cluster Headache II"; Nappi, "Case-Control Study on the Epidemiology of Cluster Headache"; Torelli et al., "Possible Predictive Factors in the Evolution of Episodic to Chronic Cluster Headache."

47. Sjaastad, Salvesen, and Antonaci, "Headache Research Strategy," 4.

48. Manzoni, "Gender Ratio of Cluster Headache over the Years," 141.

49. Rozen et al., "Cluster Headache in Women," 614.

50. Bahra, May, and Goadsby, "Cluster Headache"; Rozen and Fishman, "Female Cluster Headache in the United States of America."

51. Rozen et al., "Cluster Headache in Women"; Rozen and Fishman, "Female Cluster Headache in the United States of America."

52. See, for example, May et al., "Hypothalamic Activation in Cluster Headache Attacks."

53. Using Foucauldian genealogical methods, I trace the origin of the cluster headache profile through medical reference books on headache, making visible the process by which this construct has been created, adopted, adapted, and rejected in these canonical texts on headache. This sample was generated from all headache books shelved on the University of Michigan's medical library in 2005. Books (n=293) were identified by using the keyword "headache," in Michigan's online library database. Of these, ninety-one included some mention of cluster headache, ranging from book-length treatises (n=5) to those that devoted at least one chapter to cluster headache (n=67) to general reference books that mention cluster headaches only in passing (n=19). This sample counts multiple editions as separate books, as their content shifts between publication dates. These texts were coded for the presence or absence of the cluster profile (a full explanation of this profile appears in the analysis), crossed with the author's level of support (enthusiastic to moderate, low, reject) for various features of the cluster headache profile including its physical and psychological features and descriptions of women patients. This analysis presents a measure of authors' acceptance of the cluster profile in these headache reference books. It cannot assess authors' rationale for excluding a discussion of the cluster headache profile and therefore does not estimate the absolute number of headache experts who accept or reject this profile. Methodological approach detailed in Foucault, *Birth of the Clinic*.

54. Prince, Frader, and Bosk, "On Hedging in Physician Discourse."

55. Dodick et al., "Cluster Headache."

56. DJ's survey constitutes a type of lay epidemiology, as described by Brown, "Popular Epidemiology and Toxic Waste Contamination."

57. Connell, *Masculinities*.

58. Courtney, "Constructions of Masculinity and Their Influence on Men's Well-Being"; Harrison, "Warning"; Messner, *Politics of Masculinities*; Sabo and Gordon, *Men's Health and Illness*.

59. Fleck, *Genesis and Development of a Scientific Fact*, 38.

60. Epstein, "Bodily Differences and Collective Identities."

Conclusion

1. Schnakenberg, "Michele Bachmann News Accidentally Reveals Hidden Truths."

2. Ortega and Vidal, "Mapping the Cerebral Subject in Contemporary Culture"; Vidal, "Brainhood, Anthropological Figure of Modernity."

3. Along the lines argued by Ridgeway, *Framed by Gender*.

4. Lipton, Stewart, and Simon, "Medical Consultation for Migraine."

5. Rozen and Fishman, "Female Cluster Headache in the United States of America."

6. Armstrong, Carpenter, and Hojnacki, "Whose Deaths Matter?"; Best, "Disease Politics and Medical Research Funding."

7. Best, "Disease Politics and Medical Research Funding."

8. Ibid.

Bibliography

Books, Journals, and Websites

Abbott, Andrew. *The System of Professions: An Essay on the Division of Expert Labor*. Chicago: University of Chicago Press, 1988.

Abu-Arefeh, I., and G. Russell. "Prevalence of Headache and Migraine in Schoolchildren." *British Medical Journal* 309 (1994): 765–69.

Ackerknecht, Erwin H. "The History of Psychosomatic Medicine." *Psychological Medicine* 12 (1982): 17–24.

Ad Hoc Committee on Classification of Headache. "Classification of Headache." *Journal of the American Medical Association* 179 (1962): 717–18.

Agonito, Rosemary. *History of Ideas on Woman: A Source Book*. New York: Putnam, 1977.

Album, Dag, and Steinar Westin. "Do Diseases Have a Prestige Hierarchy? A Survey among Physicians and Medical Students." *Social Science and Medicine* 66 (2008): 182–88.

Alexander, Franz. *Psychosomatic Medicine*. New York. Norton, 1950.

Alvarez, Walter C. "The Migrainous Woman and All Her Troubles." *Alexander Blain Hospital Bulletin* 4 (1945): 3–8.

———. "Notes on the History of Migraine." *Headache* 2 (1963): 209–13.

Amin, Faisal Mohammad, Mohammad Sohail Asghar, Anders Hougaard, Adam Espe Hansen, Vibeke Andrée Larsen, Patrick J. H. de Koning, Henrik B. W. Larsson, Jes Olesen, and Messoud Ashina M. "Magnetic Resonance Angiography of Intracranial and Extracranial Arteries in Patients with Spontaneous Migraine without Aura: A Cross-Sectional Study." *Lancet Neurology* 12 (2013): 454–61.

Andrasik, F., E. B. Blanchard, and J. G. Arena. "Cross-Validation of the Kudrow-Sutkus MMPI Classification System for Diagnosing Headache Type." *Headache* 22 (1982): 2–5.

Andreasen, Nancy. *The Broken Brain: The Biological Revolution in Psychiatry*. New York: Harper and Row, 1984.

Angell, Marcia. *The Truth about Drug Companies: How They Deceive Us and What to Do about It.* New York: Random House, 2004.

Anonymous. Clusterheadaches.com. Accessed August, 27, 2013. http://clusterheadaches.com/.

Appenzeller, Otto. "No Appointment Needed; the Headache Clinic." *Headache* 11 (1971): 133.

Armstrong, Elizabeth M., Daniel P. Carpenter, and Marie Hojnacki. "Whose Deaths Matter? Mortality, Advocacy, and Attention to Disease in the Mass Media." *Journal of Health Politics, Policy and Law* 31 (2006): 729–72.

Aronowitz, Robert A. *Making Sense of Illness.* Cambridge: University of Cambridge Press, 1998.

"Atlas of Headache Disorders and Resources in the World 2011." Geneva, Switzerland: World Health Organization and Lifting the Burden, 2011.

Austen, Jane. *Sense and Sensibility.* New York: Bantam Books, 1983.

Bahra, Anish, A. May, and Peter J. Goadsby. "Cluster Headache: A Prospective Clinical Study with Diagnostic Implications." *Neurology* 58 (2002): 354–61.

Barker, Kristin. *The Fibromyalgia Story.* Philadelphia: Temple University Press, 2005.

———. "Listening to Lyrica: Contested Illnesses and Pharmaceutical Determinism." *Social Science and Medicine* 73 (2011): 833–42.

———. "Self-Help Literature and the Making of an Illness Identity: The Case of Fibromyalgia Syndrome." *Social Problems* 49 (2002): 279–300.

Barker-Benfield, G. J. *The Culture of Sensibility: Sex and Society in Eighteenth-Century Britain.* Chicago: University of Chicago Press, 1992.

Baszanger, Isabelle. *Inventing Pain Medicine: From the Laboratory to the Clinic.* New Brunswick, NJ: Rutgers University Press, 1998.

Bell, Susan E. *DES Daughters, Embodied Knowledge, and the Transformation of Women's Health Politics in the Late Twentieth Century.* Philadelphia: Temple University Press, 2009.

Bell, Susan E., and Anne E. Figert. "Gender and the Medicalization of Healthcare." In *The Palgrave Handbook of Gender and Healthcare*, edited by Ellen Kuhlmann and Ellen Annandale, 107–22. Houndsmill, Basingstoke, Hampshire, UK: Palgrave Macmillan, 2010.

Berkrot, Bill. "Global Drug Sales to Top $1 Trillion in 2014: IMS." Reuters, April 20, 2010. Accessed January 12, 2012. http://www.reuters.com/article/2010/04/20/us-pharmaceuticals-forecast-idUSTRE63J35020100420.

Bernstein, Carolyn, and Elaine McArdle. *The Migraine Brain: Your Breakthrough Guide to Fewer Headaches, Better Health.* New York: Free Press, 2008.

Bertolotti, G., G. Vidotto, E. Sanavio, and E. Frediani. "Psychological and Emotional Aspects and Pain." *Neurological Science* 24 (2003): S71–S75.

Best, Rachel Kahn. "Disease Politics and Medical Research Funding: Three Ways Advocacy Shapes Policy." *American Sociological Review* 77 (2012): 780–803.

Bigal, Marcelo E., Richard B. Lipton, Paul Winner, M. L. Reed, Seymour Diamond, and Walter F. Stewart. "Migraine in Adolescents: Association with Socioeconomic Status and Family History." *Neurology* 69 (2007): 16–25.

Binder, Amy. "Constructing Racial Rhetoric: Media Depictions of Harm in Heavy Metal and Rap Music." *American Sociological Review* 58 (1993): 753–67.

Bing, R. *Lehrbuch der Nervenkrankheiten*. Berlin: Urban and Schwarzenberg, 1913.

Blanchard, Edward B., and Frank Andrasik. *Management of Chronic Headaches: A Psychological Approach.* New York: Pergamom Press, 1985.

Blum, Linda, and Nena F. Stracuzzi. "Gender in the Prozac Nation: Popular Discourse and Productive Bodies." *Gender and Society* 18 (2004): 269–86.

Boes, C. J., D. J. Capobianco, M. S. Matharu, and P. J. Goadsby. "Wilfred Harris' Early Description of Cluster Headache." *Cephalalgia* 22 (2002): 320–26.

Bordo, Susan. *Unbearable Weight: Feminism, Western Culture, and the Body*. Berkeley: University of California Press, 1993.

Brandes, Jan L. "The Migraine Cycle: Patient Burden of Migraine during and between Migraine Attacks." *Headache* 48 (2008): 430–41.

Breslau, Naomi, Lonni Schultz, Richard Lipton, Edward Peterson, and K. M. A. Welch. "Migraine Headaches and Suicide Attempt." *Headache* 52 (2012): 723–31.

Brown, Phil. "Naming and Framing: The Social Construction of Diagnosis and Illness." *Journal of Health and Social Behavior* Special Issue (1996): 34–52.

———. "Popular Epidemiology and Toxic Waste Contamination: Lay and Professional Ways of Knowing." *Journal of Health and Social Behavior* 33 (1992): 267–81.

———. *Toxic Exposures: Contested Illnesses and the Environmental Health Movement.* New York: Columbia University Press, 2007.

Brown, Phil, Stephen Zavestoski, Sabrina McCormick, Brian Mayer, Rachel Morello-Frosch, and Rebecca Gasior Altman. "Embodied Health Movements: New Approaches to Social Movements in Health." *Sociology of Health and Illness* 26 (2004): 50–80.

Bruyn, G. W., and H. R. Weenink. "Migraine Accompagnee: A Critical Evaluation." *Headache* 6 (1966): 1–22.

Buchholz, David. *Heal Your Headache: The 1, 2, 3 Program*. New York: Workman Publishing Company, 2002.

Burwell, Bryan. "Pippen Sheds His Wimpy Image." *USA Today*, June 4, 1993.

Butler, Judith P. *Bodies That Matter: On the Discursive Limits of "Sex."* New York: Routledge, 1993.

Cady, Roger K. "Migraines and Emotional Health." *Migraine Teleconference Series.* Edited by Megan Oltman, 2009. Accessed December 7, 2013. http://freemybrain.com.

Cady, Roger K., J. K. Wendt, J. R. Kirchner, J. F. Sargent, J. F. Rothrock, and H. Skaggs. "Treatment of Acute Migraine with Subcutaneous Sumatriptan." *Journal of the American Medical Association* 165 (1991): 2831–35.

Carr, E. Summerson. "Enactments of Expertise." *Annual Review of Anthropology* 39 (2010): 17–32.

Carroll, Lewis. *Alice in Wonderland*. New York: Sam'l Gabriel Sons, 1916.

Charrett-Dykes, Catherine. "Chronic Migraine and Suicide Awareness Day." *Mindsplitters*, May 30, 2012. Accessed June 10, 2012. http://mindsplitters.blogspot.com/2012/05/chronic-migraine-and-suicide-awareness.html.

Cheyne, George. *The English Malady: Or, a Treatise of Nervous Diseases of All Kinds, as Spleen, Vapours, Lowness of Spirits, Hypochondriacal, and Hysterical Distempers*. London: Tavistock, 1733.

Clarke, Adele E., Janet K. Shim, Laura Mamo, Jennifer Ruth Fosket, and Jennifer R. Fishman. "Biomedicalization: Technoscientific Transformations of Health, Illness, and US Biomedicine." *American Sociological Review* 68 (2003): 161–94.

Collins, Lauren. "Head First." *New Yorker*, September 21, 2009. Accessed August 22, 2013. http://www.newyorker.com/talk/2009/09/21/090921ta_talk_collins.

Connell, R.W. *Masculinities*. Berkeley: University of California Press, 1995.

Conrad, Peter. "The Discovery of Hyperkinesis: Notes on the Medicalization of Deviant Behavior." *Social Problems* 23 (1975): 12–21.

———. *The Medicalization of Society: On the Transformation of Human Conditions into Treatable Disorders*. Baltimore, MD: Johns Hopkins University Press, 2007.

Conrad, Peter, and Valerie Leiter. "Medicalization, Markets and Consumers." *Journal of Health and Social Behavior* 45 (2004): 158–76.

Cooley, Charles Horton. *Human Nature and the Social Order.* New York: Scribner's, 1902.

Cooper, Lesley. "Myalgic Encephalomyelitis and the Medical Encounter." *Sociology of Health and Illness* 19 (1997): 186–207.

Corrigan, Patrick W., L. P. River, Robert K. Lundin, K. U. Wasowski, J. Campion, J. Mathison, H. Goldstein, M. Bergman, C. Gagnon, and M. A. Kubiak. "Stigmatizing Attributions about Mental Illness." *Journal of Community Psychiatry* 28 (2000): 91–102.

Couch, J. R., and C. M. Bearss. "Relief of Migraine Headache with Sexual Orgasm." *Headache* 27 (1987): 3.

Courtney, W. H. "Constructions of Masculinity and Their Influence on Men's Well-Being: A Theory of Gender and Health." *Social Science and Medicine* 50 (2000): 1385–401.

Crook, J., and E. Tunks. "Women with Pain," In *Chronic Pain: Psychosocial Factors in Rehabilitation*, edited by E. Tunks, A. Bellissimo, and R. Roy, 37–47. Malabar, FL: R. E. Krieger Publishing Company, 1990.

Curry, Philip, and Marita O'Brien. "The Male Heart and the Female Mind: A Study in the Gendering of Antidepressants and Cardiovascular Drugs in Advertisements in Irish Medical Publication." *Social Science and Medicine* 62 (2006): 1970–77.

Curtis, Pamela. "Blogger's Choice: Strange Behavior." *Make This Look Awesome*, June 15, 2012. Accessed June 16, 2012. http://makethislookawesome.blogspot.com/2012/06/nmam-bloggers-choice-strange-behavior.html.

Cutrer, F. Michael. "Functional Imaging in Primary Headache Disorders." *Headache* 48 (2008): 704–6.

Cuypers, J., H. Alternkirch, and S. Bunge. "Personality Profiles in Cluster Headache and Migraine." *Headache* 21 (1981): 21–24.

D'Alessandro, R., G. Gamberinin, G. Benassi, G. Morganti, P. Cortelli, and E. Lugaresi. "Cluster Headache in the Republic of San Marino." *Cephalalgia* 6 (1986): 159–62.

Davidoff, Robert A. *Migraine: Manifestations, Pathogenesis, and Management*. Oxford: Oxford University Press, 2002.

de Vries, Boukje, Rune R. Frants, Michel D. Ferrari, and Arn M. J. M. van den Maagdenberg. "Molecular Genetics of Migraine." *Human Genetics* 126 (2009): 115–32.

Diamond, Seymour, and Donald J. Dalessio. *The Practicing Physician's Approach to Headache*. New York: Medcom Press, 1973.

Didion, Joan. "In Bed." In *The White Album*, 168–72. New York: Simon and Schuster, 1979.

Dodick, David W., Todd D. Rozen, Peter J. Goadsby, and Stephen B. Silberstein. "Cluster Headache." *Cephalalgia* 20 (2000): 787–803.

Drexler, Madeline. "New Approaches to Neurological Pain: Planning for the Future." Report from meeting hosted by Harvard Medical School, Department of Neurology, Massachusetts General Hospital and Department of Neurology, University of California, San Francisco. Boston, MA, 2008.

Dumit, Joseph. "Illnesses You Have to Fight to Get: Facts as Forces in Uncertain, Emergent Illnesses." *Social Science and Medicine* 62 (2006): 577–90.

———. *Picturing Personhood: Brain Scans and Biomedical Identity*. Princeton, NJ: Princeton University Press, 2004.

Eadie, M. J. "An 18th Century Understanding of Migraine—Samuel Tissot (1728–1797)." *Journal of Clinical Neuroscience* 10 (2003): 414–19.

Ekbom, Karl, D. A. Svensson, H. Traff, and E. Waldenlind. "Age at Onset and Sex Ratio in Cluster Headache: Observations over Three Decades." *Cephalalgia* 22 (2002): 94–100.

Elithorn, Alick. "Migraine." *British Medical Journal* 680 (1969): 411–13.

Epstein, Steven. "Bodily Differences and Collective Identities: The Politics of Gender and Race in Biomedical Research in the United States." *Body and Society* 10 (2004): 183–204.

———. *Impure Science: AIDS, Activism, and the Politics of Knowledge*. Berkeley: University of California Press, 1996.

"Estimates of Funding for Various Research, Condition, and Disease Categories (RCDC)." National Institutes of Health, April 10, 2013. Accessed July, 6, 2013. http://report.nih.gov/categorical_spending.aspx.

Evans, R. W., R. B. Lipton, and S. D. Silberstein. "The Prevalence of Migraine in Neurologists." *Neurology* 61 (2003): 1271–72.

Evans, Sara M., and Harry C. Boyte. *Free Spaces: The Sources of Democratic Change in America*. New York: Harper and Row, 1986.

Ferrari, Michel D, Krista I. Roon, Richard B. Lipton, and Peter J. Goadsby. "Oral Triptans (Serotonin 5-Ht1b/1d Agonists) in Acute Migraine Treatment: A Meta-Analysis of 53 Trials." *Lancet* 358 (2001): 1668–75.

Finkel, Alan. "American Academic Headache Specialists in Neurology: Practice Characteristics and Culture." *Cephalalgia* 24 (2004): 522–27.

———. "The Legitimization of Headache Medicine." *Headache* 48 (2008): 711–13.

Fleck, Ludwik. *Genesis and Development of a Scientific Fact*. Chicago: University of Chicago Press, 1935/1979.

Foucault, Michel. *The Birth of the Clinic: An Archeology of Medical Perception*. New York: Vintage Books, 1963.

———. *Discipline and Punish: The Birth of the Prison*. New York: Pantheon Books, 1977.

Frank, Arthur W. *The Wounded Storyteller: Body, Illness, and Ethics*. Chicago: University of Chicago Press, 1995.

Frank, Richard, Ernst R. Berndt, Julie Donahue, Arnold Epstein, and Meredith Rosenthal. "Trends in Direct-to-Consumer Advertising of Prescription Drugs." Menlo, CA: Prepared for the Kaiser Family Foundation, 2002.

Freidson, Eliot. *Profession of Medicine: A Study of the Sociology of Applied Knowledge*. New York: Dodd, Mead, 1970.

Friedman, Arnold P. "Cluster Headaches." *Neurology* 8 (1958): 653–63.

Fujimura, Joan H. *Crafting Science: A Sociohistory of the Quest for the Genetics of Cancer*. Cambridge, MA: Harvard University Press, 1996.

Fulbright, Yvonne Kristín. "Sexpert Q&A: Sex = Headache Medicine." *Fox News Health* blog, April 7, 2009. Accessed August 10, 2013. http://health.blogs.foxnews.com/2009/04/07/sexpert-qa-sex-headache-medicine.

Furnas, Helen. "Headaches Are a Luxury." *Coronet*, March 1942, 145–49.

Gagnon, Marc-Andre, and Joel Lexchin. "The Cost of Pushing Pills: A New Estimate of Pharmaceutical Promotion Expenditures in the United States." *PLoS Medicine* 5 (2009): e1.

Galison, Peter, and Lorraine Daston. *Objectivity*. Cambridge, MA: Zone Books, 2007.

Gamson, William, and Andre Modigliani. "Media Discourse and Public Opinion on Nuclear Power." *American Journal of Sociology* 95 (1989): 1–37.

Garner, H. H., B. Shulman, P. S. MacNeal, and S. Diamond. "Psychiatric Aspects of Headache." *Headache* 7 (1967): 1–12.

Gatyas, Gary. "Modest Rise in Real Per Capita Spending; Fewer Physician Office Visits and New Therapy Starts Lead to Subdued Use of Medicines by Patient." *IMS Health*, April 19, 2011. Accessed January 12, 2012. http://www.imshealth.com/portal/site/imshealth/menuitem.a46c6d4df3db4b3d88f611019418c22a/?vgnextoid=d690a27e9d5b7210VgnVCM100000ed152ca2RCRD&vgnextfmt=default.

Geddis, Janet. "Ten Days and Counting." Migraine.com, September 24, 2006. Accessed March 16, 2012. http://migraine.com/blog/ten-days-and-counting/.

Geertz, Clifford. "Ideology as a Cultural System." In *The Interpretation of Cultures*, 193–233. New York: Basic Books, 1973.

Gieryn, Thomas F. "Boundary-Work and the Demarcation of Science from Non-Science: Strains and Interests in the Ideologies of Scientists." *American Sociological Review* 48 (1983): 781–95.

GlaxoSmithKline. "Proposed Merger of GlaxoWellcome and Smithkline Beecham: Creating the Global Leader in Pharmaceuticals." GlaxoSmithKline, January 17, 2000. Accessed September 4, 2009. http://www.gsk.com/press_archive/mrg_release_more.htm.

Goadsby, Peter J. "Pathophysiology of Cluster Headache: A Trigeminal Autonomic Cephalgia." *Lancet Neurology* 1 (2002): 251–57.

Goadsby, Peter J., Richard B. Lipton, and Michel D. Ferrari. "Migraine—Current Understanding and Treatment." *New England Journal of Medicine* 346 (2002): 257–70.

Goffman, Erving. *Gender Advertisements*. Cambridge, MA: Harvard University Press, 1979.

———. *Stigma: Notes on the Management of Spoiled Identity*. Englewood Cliffs, NJ: Prentice-Hall, 1963.

Goodell, Helen. "Thirty Years of Headache Research in the Laboratory of the Late Dr. Harold G. Wolff." *Headache* 6 (1967): 158–71.

Goodell, Helen, and Isabel Bishop Wolff. "The Influence on Medicine and Neurology of Harold G. Wolff." *Cornell University Medical College Quarterly* (Spring 1970).

Goodman, Lawrence. 2002. "Celebrity Pill Pushers." Salon.com, July 11, 2002. Accessed August 19, 2013. http://www.salon.com/2002/07/11/celebrity_drugs/.

Gowers, William R. *The Borderland of Epilepsy: Faints, Vagal Attacks, Vertigo, Migraine, Sleep Symptoms, and Their Treatment*. Philadelphia: P. Blakiston's Son, 1907.

Graham, John R. "Cluster Headache." *Headache* 11 (1972): 175–85.

Grant, Ulysses S. *Personal Memoirs of Ulysses S. Grant*. Charles L. Webster, 1885–86.

Greene, Jeremy A. *Prescribing by the Numbers: Drugs and the Definition of Illness*. Baltimore, MD: Johns Hopkins University Press, 2007.

Greenhalgh, Susan. *Under the Medical Gaze: Facts and Fiction of Chronic Pain*. Berkeley: University of California Press, 2001.

Hacking, Ian. *The Social Construction of What?* Cambridge, MA: Harvard University Press, 1999.

Hamilton, Allan McLane. *The Modern Treatment of Headaches*. Detroit, MI: George S. Davis, 1888.

Haraway, Donna. "Situated Knowledges: The Science Question in Feminism as a Site of Discourse on the Privilege of Partial Perspective." *Feminist Studies* 14 (1988): 575–99.

Harding, Sandra. *The Science Question in Feminism*. Ithaca, NY: Cornell University Press, 1986.

———. "Women's Standpoints on Nature: What Makes Them Possible?" *Osiris* 12 (1997): 186–200.

Harrison, J. "Warning: The Male Sex Role May Be Dangerous to Your Health." *Journal of Social Issues* 34 (1978): 65–86.

Harrison, Robert H. "Psychological Testing in Headache: A Review." *Headache* 14 (1975): 177–85.

Hawkins, Joellen W., and Cynthia Aber. "The Content of Advertisements in Medical Journals: Distorting the Image of Women." *Women and Health* 14 (1988): 43–59.

Hawkins, K., S. Wang, and M. Rupnow. "Direct Cost Burden among Insured US Employees with Migraine." *Headache* 48 (2008): 553–63.

Headache Classification Committee of the International Headache Society (IHS). "The International Classification of Headache Disorders, 3rd edition (beta version)." *Cephalalgia* 33 (2013): 629–808.

"Headache Disorders." *World Health Organization Fact Sheet*, March 2004. Accessed September 22, 2009. http://www.who.int/mediacentre/factsheets/fs277/en/print.html.

Hirtz, D., D. J. Thurman, K. Gwinn-Hardy, M. Mohamed, A. R. Chaudhuri, and R. Zalutsky. "How Common Are the "Common" Neurologic Disorders?" *Neurology* 68 (2007): 326–37.

Hoffman, Dianne E., and Anita J. Tarzian. "The Girl Who Cried Pain: A Bias against Women in the Treatment of Pain." *Journal of Law, Medicine and Ethics* 29 (2001): 13–27.

Hughes, Bill, and Kevin Paterson. "The Social Model of Disability and the Disappearing Body: Towards a Sociology of Impairment." *Disability and Society* 12 (1997): 325–40.

Humphrey, Patrick P. A. "The Discovery and Development of Triptans, a Major Therapeutic Breakthrough." *Headache* 48 (2008): 685–87.

Hunt, Kasie, and Molly Ball. "Michele Bachmann Faces More Migraine Questions." *Politico*, July 20, 2011. Accessed October 12, 2012. http://www.politico.com/news/stories/0711/59433.html.

Hustvedt, Siri. "Lifting, Lights and Little People." *New York Times*, February 17, 2008. Accessed February 17, 2008. http://migraine.blogs.nytimes.com/2008/02/17/lifting-lights-and-little-people/.

———. *The Shaking Woman or a History of My Nerves*. New York: Henry Holt, 2010.

Isler, Hansreudi. "Episodic Cluster Headache from a Textbook of 1745: Van Swieten's Classic Description." *Cephalalgia* 13 (1993): 172–74.

———. "The Galenic Tradition and Migraine." *Journal of the History of the Neurosciences* 1 (1992): 227–33.

Italian Cooperative Study Group on the Epidemiology of Cluster Headache. "Case-Control Study on the Epidemiology of Cluster Headache II: Anthropometric Data and Personality Profile." *Functional Neurology* 15 (2000): 215–23.

Jackson, Jean E. "'I Am a Fieldnote': Fieldnotes as a Symbol of Professional Identity." In *Fieldnotes: The Makings of Anthropology*, edited by Roger Sanjek, 3–33. Ithaca, NY: Cornell University Press, 1990.

Jordan-Young, Rebecca. *Brain Storm: The Flaws in the Science of Sex Differences*. Cambridge, MA: Harvard University Press, 2011.

Joyce, Kelly. *Magnetic Appeal: MRI and the Myth of Transparency*. Ithaca, NY: Cornell University Press, 2008.

Jutel, Annemarie Goldstein. *Putting a Name to It: Diagnosis in Contemporary Society*. Baltimore, MD: Johns Hopkins University, 2011.

Katzenstein, Mary Fainsod. "Discursive Politics and Feminist Activism in the Catholic Church." In *Feminist Organizations: Harvest of the New Women's Movement*, edited by Myra Marx Ferree, 35–52. Philadelphia: Temple University Press, 1995.

Kempner, Joanna. "A Sociologic Perspective in Migraine in Women." In *Migraine in Women*, edited by Elizabeth Loder and Dawn Marcus, 165–73. Hamilton, Ontario: BC Decker, 2003.

Kiester, Edwin. "Doctors Close in on the Mechanisms Behind Headache." *Smithsonian*, January 1987, 175–90.

Kleinman, Arthur. "Pain and Resistance: The Delegitimation and Relegitimation of Local Worlds." In *Pain as Human Experience: An Anthropological Perspective*, edited by Mary Jo Delvecchio-Good, Paul E. Brodwin, Byron J. Good, and Arthur Kleinman, 169–97. Berkeley: University of California Press, 1991.

Koehler, P.J. "Brown-Sequard's Comment on Du Bois-Reymond's 'Hemikrania Sympathicotonica.'" *Cephalalgia* 15 (1995): 370–72.

———. "Prevalence of Headache in Tulp's Observationes Medicae (1641) with a Description of Cluster Headache." *Cephalalgia* 13 (1993): 318–20.

Kommineni, Maya, and Alan G. Finkel. "Teaching Headache in America: Survey of Neurology Chairs and Residency Directors." *Headache* 45 (2005): 862–65.

Krajnak, Mark. "Glaxo Wellcome: Marketing Strategy without Bounds." *Medical Advertising News*, March 1, 1998. Accessed December 19, 2013. http://business.highbeam.com/437048/article-1G1-59875226/marketer-year-glaxo-wellcome.

Kreist, Sandra. "Engendering Pain: Discourse on the Experience of Chronic Headache in the United States." PhD diss., University of Kentucky, 1995.

Kroll-Smith, Steven, Philip M. Brown, and Valerie Gunter, eds.. *Illness and the Environment: A Reader in Contested Medicine.* New York: New York University Press, 2000.

Kudrow, Lee. *Cluster Headache: Mechanism and Management.* London: Oxford University Press, 1980.

———. "Physical and Personality Characteristics in Cluster Headache." *Headache* 13 (1974): 197–201.

———. "Plasma Testosterone Levels in Cluster Headache: Preliminary Results." *Headache* 6 (1976): 28–31.

Kudrow, Lee, and B. J. Sutkus. "MMPI Pattern Specificity in Primary Headache Disorders." *Headache* 19 (1979): 18–24.

Kunkel, Robert S. "The American Headache Society: Looking Back," *Headache* 48 (2008): 680–84.

Kunkle, E. Charles, W. Wilhoit, and L. Hamrick. "Recurrent Brief Headache in Cluster Pattern." *Transactions of the American Neurological Association* 77 (1952): 240.

Lakoff, George, and Mark Johnson. *Metaphors We Live By*. Chicago: University of Chicago Press, 1980.

Lance, James. *The Mechanism and Management of Headache.* London: Butterworths, 1969.

Lance, James W., and M. Anthony. "Some Clinical Aspects of Migraine. A Prospective Survey of 500 Patients." *Archives of Neurology* 15 (1966): 356–61.

Lance, James W., M. Anthony, and H. Hinterberger. "The Control of Cranial Arteries by Humoral Mechanisms and Its Relation to the Migraine Syndrome." *Headache* 7 (1967): 93.

Latham, Peter W. *On Nervous or Sick-Headache: Its Varieties and Treatment.* Cambridge: Deighton, Bell, 1873.

Latour, Bruno, and Steve Woolgar. *Laboratory Life: The Construction of Scientific Facts*. Princeton, NJ: Princeton University Press, 1979.

Lawrence, George Alfred. "Anteros, Chapter XXIV." *Harper's New Monthly Magazine*, November 1870.

Lee, Diana. "Finding the Right Migraine Preventive Medication Is Complicated, Frustrating." Migraine.com, April 11, 2011. Accessed April 20, 2012. http://

migraine.com/blog/finding-the-right-migraine-preventive-medication-is-complicated-frustrating/.

———. "Migraineurs: Have Happier Holidays with Routines." *Somebody Heal Me*, December 11, 2009. Accessed April 20, 2012. http://somebodyhealme.dianalee.net/2009/12/migraineurs-have-happier-holidays-with.html.

Leeloo, "Migraine and Suicide." *Healthcentral Migraine*, August 6, 2008. Accessed August 16, 2013. http://www.healthcentral.com/migraine/c/8501/37503/migraine-suicide/.

Lemos, Carolina, Isabel Alonso, José Barros, Jorge Sequeiros, José Pereira-Monteiro, Denisa Mendonça, and Alda Sousa. "Assessing Risk Factors for Migraine: Differences in Gender Transmission." *PLoS One* 7 (2012). e50626.

L'Europa, Gary A. "Stop Limiting Migraine Medicine." *Providence Journal*, June 25, 2007.

Levi, R., G.V. Edman, K. Ekbom, and E. Waldenlind. "Episodic Cluster Headache II. High Tobacco and Alcohol Consumption in Males." *Headache* 32 (1992): 184–87.

Leyton, Nevil. *Migraine and Periodic Headache: A New Approach to Successful Treatment*. London: William Heineman Medical Books, 1952.

Lichtenstein, Bill. "Migraine." *The Infinite Mind*. WNYC radio, November 12, 2001.

Lillrank, Annika. "Back Pain and the Resolution of Diagnostic Uncertainty in Illness Narratives." *Social Science and Medicine* 57 (2003): 1045–54.

Lipton, Richard B., Marcelo E. Bigal, Merle Diamond, F. Freitag, M. L. Reed, and Walter F. Stewart and on behalf of the AMPP Advisory Group. "Migraine Prevalence, Disease Burden, and the Need for Preventive Therapy." *Neurology* 68 (2007): 343–49.

Lipton, Richard B., M. E. Bigal, S. R. Rush, J. P. Yenkosky, J. N. Liberman, J. D. Bartleson, and S. D. Silberstein. "Migraine Practice Patterns among Neurologists." *Neurology* 62 (2004): 1926–31.

Lipton, Richard B., Seymour Diamond, M. Reed, Merle L. Diamond, and Walter F. Stewart. "Migraine Diagnosis and Treatment: Results from the American Migraine Study II." *Headache* 41 (2001): 638–45.

Lipton, Richard B., and Julie Pan. "Is Migraine a Progressive Brain Disease?" *Journal of the American Medical Association* 291 (2004): 493–94.

Lipton, Richard B., Walter F. Stewart, Seymour Diamond, Merle L. Diamond, and Michael Reed. "Prevalence and Burden of Migraine in the United States: Data from the American Migraine Study II." *Headache* 41 (2001): 646–57.

Lipton, Richard B., Walter F. Stewart, and David Simon. "Medical Consultation for Migraine: Results from the American Migraine Study." *Headache* 38 (1998): 87–96.

Liu, Yifei, and William R. Ducette. "Does Direct-to-Consumer Advertising Affect Patient's Choice of Pain Medication?" *Current Pain and Headache Reports* 12 (2008): 89–93.

Liveing, Edward. *On Megrim, Sick-Headache and Some Allied Disorders: A Contribution to the Pathology of Nerve-Storms*. London: J. and A. Churchill, New Burlington Street, 1873.

Livingstone, Ian, and Donna Novak. *Breaking the Headache Cycle: A Proven Program for Treating and Preventing Recurring Headaches*. New York: Henry Holt, 2004.

Loder, Elizabeth W., and S. R. Beluk. "The Influence of Gender on Evaluation and Treatment of Migraine." *Headache* 39 (1999): 366.

Lovdahl, Ulrica, Annica Riska, and Elianne Riska. "Gender Display in Scandinavian and American Advertising for Antidepressants." *Scandinavian Journal of Public Health* 27 (1999): 306–10.

Lovshin, L. L. "Clinical Caprices of Histaminic Cephalgia." *Headache* 1 (1961): 3–6.

Luhrmann, Tanya M. *Of Two Minds: The Growing Disorder in Psychiatry*. New York: Alfred A. Knopf, 2000.

Lupton, Deborah. "The Construction of Patienthood in Medical Advertising." *International Journal of Health Services* 23 (1993): 805–19.

M: The Magazine of Migraine Management. AstraZeneca Pharmaceuticals, 2001.

Mandeville, Bernard. *A Treatise of the Hypochondriack and Hysterick Diseases. In Three Dialogues.* London: J. Thonson, 1730.

Mant, Andrea, and Dorothy Broom Darroch. "Media Images and Medical Images." *Social Science and Medicine* 9 (1975): 613–18.

Manzoni, Gian C. "Gender Ratio of Cluster Headache over the Years: A Possible Role of Changes in Lifestyle." *Cephalagia* 18 (1998): 138–42.

———. "Male Preponderance of Cluster Headache Is Progressively Decreasing over the Years." *Headache* 37 (1997): 588–89.

Martin, Emily. *Flexible Bodies: Tracking Immunity in American Culture—From the Days of Polio to the Age of AIDS*. Boston: Beacon Press, 1994.

———. "Mind-Body Problems." *American Ethnologist* 27 (2000): 569–90.

———. "The Pharmaceutical Person." *Biosocieties* 1 (2006): 273–87.

———. "Talking Back to Neuro-Reductionism." In *Cultural Bodies: Ethnography and Theory*, edited by Helen Thomas and Jamilah Ahmed, 190–212. Oxford: Blackwell Press, 2004.

———. *The Woman in the Body: A Cultural Analysis of Reproduction*. Boston: Beacon Press, 1987.

May, Arne, Anish Bahra, Christian Büchel, Richard S.J. Frackowiak, and Peter J. Goadsby. "Hypothalamic Activation in Cluster Headache Attacks." *Lancet* 25 (1998): 275–78.

McNell, Liz. "Cindy McCain's Secret Struggle with Migraine." *People*, September 2, 2009. Accessed September 9, 2009. http://www.people.com/people/article/0,,20301924,00.html.

McTavish, Janice R. *Pain and Profits: The History of Headache and Its Remedies in America*. New Brunswick, NJ: Rutgers University Press, 1994.

Mease, James. *Causes, Cure, and Prevention of the Sick-Headache*. Philadelphia: Henry H. Porter, 1832.

Merskey, H., J. Brown, A. Brown, L. Malhotra, D. Morrison, and C. Ripley. "Psychological Normality and Abnormality in Persistent Headache Patients." *Pain* 23 (1985): 35–47.

Messner, Michael A. *Politics of Masculinities: Men in Movements*. Thousand Oaks, CA: Sage Publications, 1997.

Metzl, Jonathan M. *Prozac on the Couch: Prescribing Gender in the Era of Wonder Drugs*. Durham, NC: Duke University Press, 2003.

Mills, C. Wright. *The Sociological Imagination*. New York: Oxford University Press, 1959.

Morgan, Missy. "The Migraine Battle Continues." *Health Central Migraine*, December 22, 2010. Accessed June 20, 2012. http://www.healthcentral.com/migraine/c/65975/127069/battle-continues.

Morris, David B. *The Culture of Pain*. Berkeley: University of California Press, 1991.

Moss-Coane, Marty. "Radio Times." WHYY Philadelphia, July 18, 2000.

Muilenburg, Crystal. "National Headache Foundation, Healthy Women and Allergan Announce First Winner of National 'Rewrite Your Day' Educational Campaign and Contest for People Living with Chronic Migraine." Irvine, CA: Allergan, December 13, 2011.

National Center for Health Statistics. "Current Estimates from the National Health Interview Survey, 1996." Hyattsville, MD: National Institutes of Health.

Nappi, G. "Case-Control Study on the Epidemiology of Cluster Headache. I. Etiological Factors and Associated Conditions." *Neuroepidemiology* 14 (1995): 123–27.

Natoli, J. L., A. Manack, B. Dean, Q. Butler, C. C. Turkel, L. Stovner, and R. B. Lipton. "Global Prevalence of Chronic Migraine: A Systematic Review." *Cephalalgia* 30 (2010): 599–609.

Nieman, E.A., and L.J. Hurwitz. "Ocular Sympathetic Palsy in Perodic Migrainous Neuralgia." *Journal of Neurology, Neurosurgery and Psychiatry* 24 (1961): 369–73.

Noonan, Chris W., Steven J. Kathman, and Mary C. White. "Prevalence Estimates for MS in the United States and Evidence of an Increasing Trend for Women." *Neurology* 58 (2002): 136–38.

Norredam, Marie, and Dag Album. "Prestige and Its Significance for Medical Specialties and Diseases." *Scandinavian Journal of Public Health* 35 (2007): 655–61.

Okin, Susan Moller. *Women in Western Political Thought*. Princeton, NJ: Princeton University Press, 1979.

Olesen, Jes. "The International Classification of Headache Disorders." *Headache* 48 (2008): 691–93.

Olesen, Jes, I. Lekander, P. Andlin-Sobocki, and B. Jönsson. "Funding of Headache Research in Europe." *Cephalalgia* 27 (2007): 995–99.

Oltman, Megan. "It's All in Your Head." *Free My Brain*, June 19, 2008. Accessed June 20, 2012. http://freemybrain.com/its-all-in-your-head/.

Ophoff, Roel A., Gisela M. Terwindt, Monique N. Vergouwe, Ronald van Eijk, Peter J. Oefner, Susan M.G. Hoffman, Jane E. Lamerdin, Harvey W. Mohrenweiser, Dennis E. Bulman, Maurizio Ferrari, Joost Haan, Dick Lindhout, Gert-Jan B van Ommen, Marten H. Hofker, Michel D. Ferrari, and Rune R. Frants. "Familial Hemiplegic Migraine and Episodic Ataxia Type-2 Are Caused by Mutations in the Ca2+ Channel Gene Cacn11a4." *Cell* 87 (1994): 543–52.

Ortega, Francisco, and Fernando Vidal. "Mapping the Cerebral Subject in Contemporary Culture." *Reciis: Electronic Journal of Communication, Information and Communication in Health* 1 (2007): 255–59.

Osterweis, Marian, Arthur Kleinman, and David Mechanic, eds. *Pain and Disability: Clinical, Behavioral, and Public Policy Perspectives*. Washington, DC: National Academy Press, 1987.

Packard, Russell C. "Psychiatric Aspects of Headache." *Headache* 19 (1979): 168–72.

Parsons, Talcott. "Social Structure and Dynamic Process: The Case of Modern Medical Practice." In *The Social System*, 428–79. New York: The Free Press, 1951.

Pearce, J. M. S. "Edward Liveing's (1832–1919) Theory of Nerve-Storms in Migraine." In *A Short History of Neurology: The British Contribution 1660–1910*, edited by F. Clifford Rose, 117–31. Oxford: Butterworth Heinemann, 1999.

Pescosolido, Bernice A., Jack K. Martin, J. Scott Long, Tait R. Medina, Jo C. Phelan, and Bruce G. Link. "'A Disease Like Any Other'? A Decade of Change in Public Reactions to Schizophrenia, Depression, and Alcohol Dependence." *American Journal of Psychiatry* 167 (2010): 1321–30.

Petryna, Adriana. *Life Exposed: Biological Citizens after Chernobyl*. Princeton, NJ: Princeton University Press, 2002.

Pfaffenrath, Volker, Josef Hummelsberger, Walter Pöllman, Holder Kaube, and Michael Rath. "MMPI Personality Profiles in Patients with Primary Headache Syndromes." *Cephalalgia* 11 (1991): 263–68.

"Pfizer Gives Its New Relpax Drug the Spa Treatment." *Medical Marketing and Media* 38 (2003): 18.

Phelan, Jo. "Geneticization of Deviant Behavior and Consequences for Stigma: The Case of Mental Illness." *Journal of Health and Social Behavior* 46 (2005): 307–22.

Phillips, Pat. "Migraine as a Woman's Issue—Will Research and New Treatments Help?" *Journal of the American Medical Association* 280 (1998): 1975–76.

Pines, Wayne L. "A History and Perspective on Direct-to-Consumer Promotion." *Food and Drug Law Journal* 54 (1999): 489–518.

Plato. *Charmides*. Stockbridge, MA: Hard Press, 2006.

Porter, Theodore M. *Trust in Numbers: The Pursuit of Objectivity in Science and Public Life*. Princeton, NJ: Princeton University Press, 1996.

Prather, Jane, and Linda S. Fidell. "Sex Differences in the Content and Style of Medical Advertisements." *Social Science and Medicine* 9 (1975): 23–26.

Prince, Ellen, Joel Frader, and Charles L. Bosk. "On Hedging in Physician Discourse: Proceedings of the Second Annual Delaware Symposium on Language Studies." In *Linguistics and the Professions*, edited by R. J. DiPietro, 83–97. Norwood, NJ: Ablex Publishing, 1982.

Rabinow, Paul. "Artificiality and Enlightenment: From Sociobiology to Biosociality." In *Essays on the Anthropology of Reason*, 91–111. Princeton, NJ: Princeton University Press, 1996.

Rapoport, Alan M., Fred D. Sheftell, and Stewart J. Tepper. *Conquering Headache*. Hamilton, London: Decker DTC, 2003.

Raskin, Neil. "Conclusions." *Headache* 30 (1990): 24–28.

Reilly, Thomas F. *Headache: Its Causes and Treatment*. Philadelphia: P. Blakiston's Sons, 1926.

Richardson, Sarah. "Sexing the X: How the X Became the 'Female Chromosome.'" *Signs* 37 (2012): 909–33.

Ridgeway, Cecilia. *Framed by Gender: How Gender Inequality Persists in the Modern World*. Oxford: Oxford University Press, 2011.

Riska, Elianne. "Gender and Medicalization and Biomedicalization Theories." In *Biomedicalization: Technoscience, Health, and Illness in the U.S.*, edited by Adele E. Clarke, Laura Mamo, Jennifer Ruth Fosket, Jennifer R. Fishman, and Janet K. Shim, 147–52. Durham, NC: Duke University Press, 2010.

———. *Masculinity and Men's Health: Coronary Heart Disease in Medical and Public Discourse*. Lanham, MD: Rowman and Littlefield, 2004.

Robert, Teri. "Defeated, Hopeless, Powerless, Useless—Migraine in a Word." Migraine.com, October 6, 2011. Accessed August 8. 2012. http://migraine.com/blog/defeated-hopeless-powerless-useless-migraine-in-a-word/.

———. "Elvis and LSD? No, DHE for Migraine! Elvis Presley's Private Struggle with Intractable Migraines Revealed." About.com, June 12, 2006. Accessed June 20. 2012 http://headaches.about.com/cs/profiles/a/elvis_mig.htm.

———. *Living Well with Migraine Disease and Headaches: What Your Doctor Doesn't Tell You . . . That You Need to Know*. New York: William Morrow, 2005.

———. "Migraine Research Funding—An Important Step." *Health Central Migraine*, May 23, 2010. Accessed July 6, 2012. http://www.healthcentral.com/migraine/c/123/112308/research-important/.

———. "Re: Understanding Migraine Disease and Migraineurs. *Help for Headaches and Migraine*. Accessed December 12, 2013. http://www.helpforheadaches.com/lwfiles/family-mig-letter.htm.

———. "10 Things I Want to Share about Migraines." Migraine.com, November 22, 2011. Accessed July 6, 2012. http://migraine.com/blog/10-things-i-want-to-share-about-migraines/.

Robinson, Michael E., Michael E. Geisser, John N. Dieter, and Bernard Swerdlow. "The Relationship between MMPI Cluster Membership and Diagnostic Category in Headache Patients." *Headache* 31 (1991): 111–15.

Rose, Nikolas. *The Politics of Life Itself: Biomedicine, Power, and Subjectivity in the Twenty-First Century.* Princeton, NJ: Princeton University Press, 2007.

Rose, Nikolas, and Carlos Novas. "Biological Citizenship." In *Global Assemblages: Technology, Politics, and Ethics as Anthropological Problems*, edited by Aihwa Ong and Stephen J. Collier, 439–63. Oxford: Oxford University Press, 2005.

Rosen, N. L. and E. Mauser. "So Many Migraines, So Few Specialists: Analysis Of The Geographic Location Of United Council For Neurologic Subspecialties (UCNS) Certified Headache Specialists Compared To USA Headache Demographics." *Cephalalgia* 33 (2013): 146–47.

Rosenberg, Charles E. "Body and Mind in Nineteenth-Century Medicine: Some Clinical Origins of the Neurosis Construct." *Bulletin of the History of Medicine* 63 (1989): 185–97.

———. "Contested Boundaries: Psychiatry, Disease and Diagnosis." *Perspectives in Biology and Medicine* 49 (2006): 407–24.

———. "The Tyranny of Diagnosis: Specific Entities and Individual Experience." *Milbank Quarterly* 80 (2002): 237–60.

Rosenberg, Charles E., and Janet Golden, Eds. *Framing Disease: Studies in Cultural History*. New Brunswick, NJ: Rutgers University Press, 1992.

Ross, James. *A Treatise on the Diseases of the Nervous System*. London: J and A Churchill, New Burlington Street, 1881.

Rothrock, John F. "In This Issue." *Headache* 48 (2008): 669.

Rozen, Todd D., and R. S. Fishman. "Female Cluster Headache in the United States of America: What Are the Gender Differences? Results from the United States Cluster Headache Survey." *Journal of the Neurological Sciences* 317 (2012): 17–28.

Rozen, Todd D., R. M. Niknam, A. L. Shechter, William B. Young, and Stephen D. Silberstein. "Cluster Headache in Women: Clinical Characteristics and Comparison with Cluster Headaches in Men." *Journal of Neurology, Neurosurgery and Psychiatry* 70 (2001): 613–17.

Ruiz de Velasco, I., N. Gonzalez, Y. Etxeberria, and J. C. Garcia-Monco. "Quality of Life in Migraine Patients: A Qualitative Study." *Cephalalgia* 23 (2003): 892–900.

Rush, Ladonna L. "Affective Reactions to Multiple Social Stigmas." *Journal of Social Psychology* 138 (1998): 421–30.

Sabo, D., and D. F. Gordon, eds. *Men's Health and Illness: Gender, Power, and the Body*. Thousand Oaks, CA: Sage Publications, 1995.

Sacks, Oliver. *Migraine: Revised and Expanded*. New York: Vintage Books, 1970/1992.

———. "Patterns." *New York Times*, February 13, 2008. Accessed February 13, 2008. http://migraine.blogs.nytimes.com/2008/02/13/patterns/.

Sahoo, Alison. *Lifecycle Management Strategies: Maximizing ROI through Indication Expansion, Reformulation and RX-to-OTC Switching*. Business Insights, 2006.

Saper, Joel R. *Headache Disorders: Current Concepts and Treatment Strategies*. Boston: J. Wright PSG, 1983.

———. "Nonheadache Disorders and Characteristics of Cluster Headache Patients." In *Cluster Headache*, edited by Ninan T. Mathew, 31–44. Jamaica, NY: Spectrum Publications, 1984.

Saper, Joel R., and Kenneth R. Magee. *Freedom from Headaches: A Personal Guide for Understanding and Treating Headache, Face, and Neck Pain*. New York: Simon and Schuster, 1978.

Scarry, Elaine. *The Body in Pain: The Making and Unmaking of the World*. New York: Oxford University Press, 1985.

Scher, Ann I., Walter F. Stewart, Joshua Liberman, and Richard B. Lipton. "Prevalence of Frequent Headache in a Population Sample." *Headache* 38 (1998): 497–506.

Schiebinger, Londa L. *The Mind Has No Sex? Women in the Origins of Modern Science*. Cambridge, MA: Harvard University Press, 1989.

Schiller, F. "Prophylactic and Other Treatment for 'Histaminic Cluster' or Limited Variant of Migraine." *Journal of the American Medical Association* 173 (1960): 1907–11.

Schnakenberg, Ellen. "Michele Bachmann News Accidentally Reveals Hidden Truths." Migraine.com, July 22, 2011. Accessed October 11, 2012. http://migraine.com/blog/michele-bachmann-news-accidentally-reveals-hidden-truths/?comments=.

———. "Migraine and the ER—a Follow-Up Interview." Migraine.com, February 8, 2012. Accessed June 18, 2012. http://migraine.com/blog/expert-featured-article/migraine-the-er-%E2%80%93-a-follow-up-interview/.

———. "The Migraine Dirty Dozen—Things Not to Say to a Chronic Migraineur." Migraine.com, January 10, 2012. Accessed June 15, 2012. http://migraine.com/blog/living-with-migraine/the-migraine-dirty-dozen-things-not-to-say-to-a-chronic-migraineur.

———."Migraine Milestones: Exciting Announcements for Patients." Migraine.com, June 28, 2012. Accessed August 26, 2013. http://migraine.com/blog/migraine-milestones-exciting-announcements-for-patients/.

———. "Why Does the Emergency Room Treat Me like a Drug Seeker?" Migraine.com, December 7, 2011. Accessed June 8, 2012. http://migraine.com/blog/living-with-migraine/why-does-the-emergency-department-treat-me-like-a-drug-seeker/.

———. "Why Is Migraine Capitalized?" Migraine.com, February 27, 2012. Accessed June 10, 2012. http://migraine.com/blog/living-with-migraine/why-is-migraine-capitalized/.

Schneider, Joseph W., and Peter Conrad. "In the Closet with Illness: Epilepsy, Stigma Potential and Information Control." *Social Problems* 28 (1980): 32–44.

Schudson, Michael. "How Culture Works: Perspectives from Media Studies on the Efficacy of Symbols." *Theory and Society* 18 (1989): 153–80.

Schürks, Markus, Pamela M. Rist, Marcelo E. Bigal, Julie E. Buring, Richard B. Lipton, and Tobias Kurth. "Migraine and Cardiovascular Disease: Systematic Review and Meta-Analysis." *British Medical Journal* 339 (2009): b3914.

Schwendt, Todd J., and Robert E. Shapiro. "Funding of Research on Headache Disorders by the National Institutes of Health." *Headache* 49 (2009): 162–69.

Scott, Joan W. "Gender: A Useful Category of Historical Analysis." *American Historical Review* 91 (1986): 1053–75.

Segal, Judy Z. *Health and the Rhetoric of Medicine*. Carbondale: Southern Illinois University Press, 2005.

Selinsky, H. "Psychologic Study of the Migrainous Syndrome." *Bulletin of the New York Academy of Medicine* 15 (1939): 757–63.

Shapiro, Robert E., and Peter J. Goadsby. "The Long Drought: The Dearth of Public Funding for Headache Research." *Cephalalgia* 27 (2007): 991–94.

Sheftell, Fred D., and Stewart J. Tepper. "New Paradigms in the Recognition and Acute Treatment of Migraine." *Headache* 41 (2002): 58–69.

Sicuteri, F. "Prophylactic and Therapeutic Properties of Methyl Lysergic Acid Butanolamide in Migraine." *International Archives of Allergy* 15 (1959): 300.

Silberstein, Stephen, "Ergotamine and Dihydroergotamine: History, Pharmacology, and Efficacy." *Headache* 43 (2003): 144–66.

Silberstein, Stephen, Richard B. Lipton, and Peter J. Goadsby. *Headache in Clinical Practice*. London: Martin Dunitz, 2002.

Silberstein, Stephen, Elizabeth Loder, Seymour Diamond, M. L. Reed, Marcelo E. Bigal, and Richard B. Lipton. "Probable Migraine in the United States: Results of the American Migraine Prevalence and Prevention (AMPP) Study." *Cephalalgia* 27 (2007): 220–29.

Silberstein, Stephen, and John Rothrock, eds. *The State of Migraine: Prevention and Treatment*. Arlington Heights, IL: Access Medical Group, 2002.

Silverman, Chloe. *Understanding Autism: Patients, Doctors, and the History of the Disorder*. Princeton, NJ: Princeton University Press, 2013.

Simonds, Wendy, Barbara Katz Rothman, and Bari Meltzer Norman. *Laboring On: Birth in Transition in the United States*. New York: Routledge, 2006.

Sismondo, Sergio. "Ghost Management: How Much of the Medical Literature Is Shaped behind the Scenes by the Pharmaceutical Industry?" *PLoS Medicine* 4 (2007): e286.

Sjaastad, Ottar. *Cluster Headache Syndrome*. London: W. B. Saunders, 1992.

Sjaastad, Ottar, R. Salvesen, and F. Antonaci. "Headache Research Strategy." *Cephalalgia* 7 (1987): 1–6.

Sjoberg, Gideon, Norma Williams, Ted R. Vaughan, and Andree F. Sjoberg. "The Case Study Approach in Social Research: Basic Methodological Issues." In *The Case for the Case Study*, edited by Anthony M. Orum, Joe R. Feagin, and Gideon Sjoberg, 27–79. Chapel Hill: University of North Carolina Press, 1991.

Smith, Dorothy. *The Conceptual Practices of Power: A Feminist Sociology of Knowledge*. Boston: Northeastern University Press, 1990.

Smyres, Kerrie. "The Day-to-Day Life of a Chronic Migraineur." *The Daily Headache*, January 20, 2012. Accessed June 15, 2012. http://www.thedailyheadache.com/2012/01/the-day-to-day-life-of-a-chronic-migraineur.html.

———. "Not Just a Headache: Migraine's Other Symptoms." *The Daily Headache*, December 19. 2005. Accessed August 26, 2013. http://www.thedailyheadache.com/2005/12/other_symptoms_.html.

———. "Requesting Accommodations Eases Burden of Disability." Migraine.com, April 27, 2012. Accessed June 15, 2012. http://migraine.com/blog/living-with-migraine/requesting-accommodations-eases-burden-of-disability/.

Somers, Margaret. "The Narrative Constitution of Identity: A Relational and Network Approach." *Theory and Society* 23 (1994): 605–49.

Sontag, Susan. *Illness as Metaphor and AIDS and Its Metaphors*. New York: Picador, 2001.

South, Valerie, and Fred Sheftell. "Communicating with the Patient." In *Wolff's Headache and Other Head Pain*, edited by Stephen D. Silberstein, Richard B. Lipton, and Donald J. Dalessio, 599–606. New York: Oxford University Press, 2001.

Spanier, Bonnie. *Im/Partial Science: Gender Ideology in Molecular Biology*. Bloomington: Indiana University Press, 1995.

Sprague, Joey, and Mary K. Zimmerman. "Overcoming Dualisms: A Feminist Agenda for Sociological Methodology." In *Theory on Gender/Feminism On Theory*, edited by Paula England, 255–79. New York: Aldine DeGruyter, 1993.

Steinem, Gloria. "If Men Could Menstruate." *Ms. Magazine*, October 1978.

Stewart, Walter F., J. A. Ricci, E. Chee, D. Morganstein, and R. B. Lipton. "Lost Productive Time and Cost Due to Common Pain in the US Workforce." *Journal of the American Medical Association* 290 (2003): 2443–54.

Stewart, Walter F., D. Simon, A. Shechter, and Richard B. Lipton. "Population Variation in Migraine Prevalence: A Meta-Analysis." *Journal of Clinical Epidemiology* 48 (1995): 269–80.

"Stink over Perfume at Detroit Workplace." *CBS News*, March 30, 2010. Accessed August 23, 2013. http://www.cbsnews.com/stories/2010/03/16/earlyshow/main6303548.shtml.

Strong, Jonathan. "Stress-Related Condition 'Incapacitates' Bachmann; Heavy Pill

Use Alleged." *Daily Caller*, July 18, 2011. Accessed October 12, 2012. http://dailycaller.com/2011/07/18/stress-related-condition-incapacitates-bachmann-heavy-pill-use-alleged/—ixzz291R52W1G:

Swidler, Ann. "Culture in Action: Symbols and Strategies." *American Sociological Review* 51 (1986): 273–86.

Symonds, John Addington. "The Gulstonian Lectures at the Royal College of Physicians." *Medical Times and Gazette* (1848).

"Tea for Two or the World Is My Teacup." *Girl Interpreted*, June 3, 2012. Accessed August 26, 2013. http://prosetrail12.tumblr.com/post/24349060033/tea-for-two-or-the-world-is-my-teacup.

Torelli, P., D. Cologno, C. Cademartiri, and G. C. Manzoni. "Possible Predictive Factors in the Evolution of Episodic to Chronic Cluster Headache." *Headache* 40 (2000): 798–808.

Treichler, Paula. *How to Have Theory in an Epidemic: Cultural Chronicle of AIDS.* Durham, NC: Duke University Press, 1999.

Troyer, Lisa. "Legitimacy." In *Blackwell Encyclopedia of Sociology Online*, edited by George Ritzer. Accessed September 6, 2013. http://www.sociologyencyclopedia.com/public/tocnode?id=g9781405124331_yr2012_chunk_g978140512433118_ss1-29.

Tweedy, Jeff. "Shaking It Off." *New York Times*, March 5, 2008. Accessed June 12, 2013. migraine.blogs.nytimes.com/2008/03/05/shaking-it-off/.

Valendy, Jamie. "Elevator Blog," November 14, 2011. Accessed August 26, 2013. http://www.chronicmigrainewarrior.com/2011/11/elevator-blog.html.

Vidal, Fernando. "Brainhood, Anthropological Figure of Modernity." *History of the Human Sciences* 22 (2009): 5–36.

Vrettos, Athena. *Somatic Fictions: Imagining Illness in Victorian Culture*. Stanford, CA: Stanford University Press, 1995.

Wahle, Kelly. "Five Things That Changed My Life." *Living With Hope*, November 5, 2011. Accessed June 18, 2012. http://www.flywithhope.com/2011/11/five-things-that-changed-my-life.html.

Wailoo, Keith. *Dying in the City of the Blues: Sickle Cell Anemia and the Politics of Race and Health.* Chapel Hill: University of North Carolina Press, 2001.

Ware, Norma C. "Suffering and the Social Construction of Illness: The Delegitimation of Illness Experience in Chronic Fatigue Syndrome." *Medical Anthropology Quarterly* 6 (1992): 347–61.

Waters, W. E., and P. J. O'Connor. "Epidemiology of Headache and Migraine in Women." *Journal of Neurology, Neurosurgery and Psychiatry* 34 (1971): 148–53.

Weber, Mike. "Pippen Picks Horrible Time For a Headache." *Sporting News*, June 11, 1990, 38.

Weiner, Bernard, R. P. Perry, and J. Magnusson. "An Attributional Analysis of Reactions to Stigmas." *Journal of Personality and Social Psychology* 55 (1988): 738–48.

Werner, Anne, and Kristi Malterud. "It Is Hard Work Behaving as a Credible Patient: Encounters between Women with Chronic Pain and Their Doctors." *Social Science and Medicine* 57 (2003): 1409–19.

Wessman, Maija, Gisela M. Terwindt, Mari A. Kaunisto, and Roel A. Ophoff. "Migraine: A Complex Genetic Disorder." *Lancet Neurology* 6 (2007): 521–32.

"What Causes Migraine Headaches?" Health Talk Webcast, February 21, 2007. Accessed May 16, 2008. www.healthtalk.com/migraine/programs/28_706/index.cfm?pview=rpl.

Whelan, Emma. "'No One Agrees except for Those of Us Who Have It': Endometriosis Patients as an Epistemological Community." *Sociology of Health and Illness* (2007): 957–82.

Whittaker, Rosemary. "Re-Framing the Representation of Women in Advertisements for Hormone Replacement Therapy." *Nursing Inquiry* 5 (1998): 77–86.

Wilbon, Michael. "Pippen, Bulls Were out of It." *Washington Post*, June 4, 1990.

Williams, Simon. J., Jonathan Gabe, and Peter Davis. "The Sociology of Pharmaceuticals: Progress and Prospects." *Sociology of Health and Illness* 30 (2008): 813–24.

Williams, Simon J., Paul Martin, and Jonathan Gabe. "The Pharmaceuticalisation of Society? A Framework for Analysis." *Sociology of Health and Illness* 33 (2011): 719–25.

Willis, Thomas. *The London Practice of Physick: Or the Whole Practical Part of Physick Contained in the Works of Dr. Willis. Faithfully Made English, and Printed Together for the Publick Good.* London: Thomas Basset and William Crooke, 1685.

Wolff, Harold G. *Headache and Other Head Pain*, 2nd ed. New York: Oxford University Press, 1963.

———. *Stress and Disease*. Springfield, IL: Thomas, 1953.

Wolff, Harold G., and Stewart Wolf. *Pain*. Springfield, IL: Thomas, 1948.

Young, William B., Joanna Kempner, Elizabeth W. Loder, Jason Roberts, Judy Z. Segal, Miriam Solomon, Roger K. Cady, Laura Janoff, Robert D. Sheeler, Teri Robert, Jennifer Yocum, and Fred D. Sheftell. "Naming Migraine and Those Who Have It." *Headache* 52 (2012): 283–91.

Young, William B., Iris X. Tian, Jung E. Park, Joanna Kempner. "The Stigma of Migraine." *PLoS One* 8 (2013). e54074.

Zanitsch, Heather. "Stop the Insanity." *The Journey of a Migraineur*, February 8, 2008. Accessed June 18. 2012. http://aloofelf.blogspot.com/.

Zborowski, Mark. *People in Pain.* San Francisco: Jossey-Bass, 1969.

Archives

Harold G. Wolff papers. 1922–1970a. New York Weill Cornell Medical Center Archives, New York, NY.

Index

Page numbers followed by *f* indicate a figure. Those followed by *t* indicate a table.

www.ingramcontent.com/pod-product-compliance
Lightning Source LLC
Chambersburg PA
CBHW032128020426
42334CB00016B/1075

* 9 7 8 0 2 2 6 1 7 9 1 5 5 *